THE ART OF REFLEXOLOGY

Inge Dougans was born in Denmark where she also received her reflexology training. In 1981 she moved to South Africa where she set up her own clinic. In 1983 she started the School of Reflexology and Meridian Therapy and in 1985 she formed the South African Reflexology Society. She gives lectures and workshops on reflexology throughout the UK, Europe and the USA and runs a busy practice in South Africa.

Suzanne Ellis was born in South Africa. She obtained an English degree from the University of Natal and has worked as a journalist, documentary script-writer and magazine editor. She trained as a reflexologist with Inge Dougans.

THE ART OF
REFLEXOLOGY

A New Approach Using the Chinese Meridian Theory

INGE DOUGANS

with

SUZANNE ELLIS

ELEMENT
Shaftesbury, Dorset ● Rockport, Massachusetts
Brisbane, Queensland

© Inge Dougans with Suzanne Ellis 1992

First published in Great Britain in 1992 by
Element Books Limited
Shaftesbury, Dorset SP7 8BP

Published in the USA in 1992 by
Element Books, Inc.
PO Box 830, Rockport, MA 01966

Published in Australia in 1992 by
Element Books Limited for
Jacaranda Wiley Limited
33 Park Road, Milton, Brisbane 4064

Reprinted 1992
Reprinted August and December 1993
Reprinted March and September 1994
Reprinted February, April and September 1995

Cover illustration by Max Fairbrother
based on an illustration © Inge Dougans
Cover design by Max Fairbrother
Illustration by Taurus Graphics
Text design and DTP by
Pete Russell, Faringdon, Oxfordshire
Keyboarding by Poole Typesetting (Wessex) Ltd.
Printed and bound in the USA by
RR Donnelley & Sons

British Library Cataloguing in Publication
Data available

Library of Congress Cataloging in Publication
Data available

ISBN 1–85230–236–4

Preface

My career in reflexology started unexpectedly. It came about as a result of the desire to have children. For two years I had attempted, unsuccessfully, to conceive. My medical practitioner at the time in Denmark diagnosed blocked fallopian tubes. He said my only option was an operation which had a 10–15% chance of success. I decided on the operation. My mother intervened, and suggested I try a reflexologist first. I was sceptical. How could reflexology afford me the opportunity of falling pregnant, when the reputable medical profession believed there to be only a minor possibility? However, I reluctantly agreed to give it a try . . . and after the second of ten treatments, I conceived. Today I am the proud mother of two wonderful boys – who have had to accept as a mother, a career woman with a time-consuming interest and involvement in the practice and development of reflexology as an important and reputable complementary healing art. Which sometimes means they have to do without me more than they, or I, would like, but without reflexology they would possibly never have come into my life.

Reflexology has enlightened me as to the tremendously important role feet play in health and well–being, and of the tales feet can tell about the state of the body. I had, prior to reflexology treatment, suffered from extremely painful, sensitive, cracked heels. They were sometimes so itchy that I picked them till they were raw, which made walking unpleasantly painful. As you will learn from this book, the heels represent the pelvic area – and this was where I suffered severe congestion. During my course of reflexology treatment, the condition of my heels gradually improved until they were completely healed, and no longer troubled me. This of course coincided with the healing of my fallopian tubes.

I have now been a practising reflexologist for ten years, and have taught reflexology for 8 years. Over the years of practising, and listening carefully to clients' complaints, it became obvious to me that there had to be a link between the meridians described in Chinese acupuncture, and reflexology; that one should understand the body in terms of energy, realize that an unimpeded energy circulation is essential to health, and perceive disease as the result of congestions in ch'i energy. These congestions can be caused by numerous factors, but most importantly, negative attitudes, incorrect diet and breathing, and the modern enemies, stress, and electromagnetic and environmental pollution. Careful study of the feet, foot problems and the meridians convinced me that the presence of meridians in the feet had a great deal to do with the efficacy of reflexology. This book evolved as I felt it was time to share the knowledge I have accumulated over the years, and to introduce a new aspect to reflexology – an aspect which will hopefully serve to expand, and enhance, complementary therapies.

This book is dedicated to my mother, Mary Andersen, who convinced me to seek reflexology treatment; to my husband Patrick and my two sons Daniel and Thomas for giving me the support and freedom I need to enable me to teach and practise reflexology; and to my students who have helped make it all worth while. Thank you.

Also thanks to Orla Duedahl from ConTime Video Production who produced and directed the video, *The Art of Reflexology*, as a practical illustration to the book.

A special thanks must go to one of my advanced students, Suzanne Ellis who undertook the very special task of compiling all this knowledge. Without her this book would still be a dream.

Inge Dougans
Durban, South Africa

Foreword

CHRISTINE ISSEL

There is no one correct theory on how reflexology works. What is agreed by all reflexologists, regardless of the techniques they employ or the theory they believe in, is:

1. that the body is reflected on the feet through a system of reflexes; and

2. the objective of the reflexologist is to stimulate these reflexes.

It is always refreshing and stimulating to find a book on new theories regarding reflexology instead of one which restates old ideas. Inge Dougans' thesis does not contradict existing works in the field. Instead it reinforces what we have been taught through conventional anatomy and physiology. *The Art of Reflexology* provides practical and simple to use techniques for applying reflexology. Then it goes further in expanding our horizons through the presentation of a new theory based on meridians, and a new method of applying pressure to the feet via the VacuFlex system.

Every field of endeavour, including reflexology, requires constant research, development and growth. I am very excited about *The Art of Reflexology* because it introduces a new depth to the body of knowledge which comprises the profession. In her work, Inge Dougans joins East and West. First she takes the mystery out of Chinese traditional medicine and the meridians. Then she ties the Eastern concept of meridians to the Western concept of the electromagnetism of the body as put forth by Dr Robert Becker. Since the electromagnetism of the body has been scientifically established and documented, this should make the relationship of the reflexes to the meridians more acceptable to the Western mind.

Professional reflexologists owe it to their clients and themselves to investigate, with an open mind, any theories and techniques which produce results. They should study them objectively, apply the techniques themselves and then form a judgement based on their own experience. I encourage every student of reflexology, whether novice or expert, to make *The Art of Reflexology* an addition to his library, to read it with an open mind, and then decide for himself the validity of the concepts put forth by Inge Dougans.

C. I.
Sacramento, California

Endorsement

DR LESLIE F. PLEASS ND, DO, D.HOM, FSAHA

Over the years I have grown to respect Inge Dougans for utilizing her trust and belief in reflexology with her ability to teach, instruct and inspire. It is therefore a great pleasure for me to recommend her book to people who wish to care for others through the art and science of reflexology. A new breed of reflexologists is emerging – reflexologists better able to understand the workings of the human body. The upgrading of the standard of reflexology through people such as Inge Dougans will help them to work and bond well with other alternative therapies. The science of reflexology, like many 'alternatives' to modern medicine, is not fully explained to the satisfaction of science. But the art of its application has numerous consumers satisfied with its positive effects.

The VacuFlex reflexology system developed and taught by Inge Dougans, has certainly expanded the realm of reflexology. Use of the 'boot' and cupping is a useful adjunct to any healing discipline. With the VacuFlex system it is possible to pinpoint problem areas in the body, but it should be used purely as a guideline, not a diagnostic tool.

The concept of reflexology expressed in this book has a major advantage over other systems of reflexology. The combination of the two concepts of reflexology and acupuncture meridians creates a harmonious blend allowing explanation and application of knowledge in a rational and relevant fashion. The interface of these two therapies will encourage reflexologists to rise to new levels of clinical competence.

In acupuncture, the energy circulation of the body has various protective functions – to protect the body from inherent disruption and from external disruption. Reflexology and the VacuFlex system are most effective on the meridians of the body. Acupuncture meridians, first discovered many thousands of years ago, describe a system of energy that flows throughout the body providing protection to the inner mechanisms of the body. Acupuncturists, like many other complementary/alternative therapists, share the opinion that the body is a vitalistic self-curing mechanism, given the right environment and stimuli. Reflexology, by stimulating the feet, encourages positive changes throughout the body, by stimulating the body's own healing potential. The fact that major acupuncture meridians pass through the feet, makes even more valid the stimulation of the feet for therapeutic effect.

This book covers all the basics of reflexology, and also includes fascinating sections such as the mythology of feet, and problems that affect the feet, for example bunions and callouses, and their clinical meaning in terms of the meridians. The meridians and reflexes of the feet are clearly and fully discussed and illustrated. Related muscle problems are also discussed, and this integration of applied kinesiology to the feet is, I believe, also unique.

This book would therefore be of great benefit to any person wishing to learn more about the art and science of reflexology.

L.F.P.
Editor of the
Wholistic Practitioner

Contents

Author's Special Note

Throughout this book, the term 'foot massage' is used as a convenient shorthand to describe reflexology. However, the authors would stress that this is a convenience term only and is not a proper technical description of the therapy. Reflexology is not massage as understood in the systematic and scientific manipulation of the soft tissues of the body. Reflexology is the application of specific pressures to reflex points in the hands and feet. Nevertheless we feel massage is useful shorthand justified in this instance for a general understanding of what is involved.

Section one

INTRODUCTION

IN the last few decades, reflexology has evolved into a respected and effective healing art. The success of this therapy is the result of the work of dedicated practitioners worldwide. As time progresses, so does reflexology. Continued practice, study, research and awareness open new doors in the development of this therapy. The object of this book is to do just that – to open new doors in order to advance and enhance the practice of reflexology. This book differs from the majority of reflexology books available today in that it incorporates the ancient Chinese concept of meridian therapy as an important and effective adjunct to reflexology.

Both zone therapy (to date, the primary basis of reflexology study) and meridian therapy are based on the premise that energy channels or pathways traverse throughout the body, linking organs and body parts. The efficacy of reflexology is believed to be the result of stimulating and revitalizing this energy flow. Thus it is necessary to have some concept of the fascinating phenomenon – energy.

Energy is the basis of all life and a vital factor in healing. As reflexologists we are primarily concerned with internal body energy. This is examined mainly in the light of the Chinese medical system, but a brief look at the work of some modern scientists on the energy theory is also incorporated. A more comprehensive knowledge of energy will enhance one's understanding of the interconnectedness of all things in the universe. This, in turn, will promote better comprehension of the holistic health philosophy – a philosophy of prime importance to anyone intending to study and practise reflexology.

In traditional Eastern medical systems – notably the Chinese healing system and the Indian Ayurvedic system – it has long been accepted that health is based on the harmonious flow of energies. These systems believe that an intricate realm of subtle energy flows permeate the universe and that the physical, material world is but a gross manifestation of these energies. In the West, however, this concept has been difficult to accept, based 'only' on thousands of years of successful application in Eastern healing practices. Locked within the blinkered confines of conventional medicine, Westerners are obsessive about 'scientific proof' – an obsession which has, for far too long, effectively undermined many invaluable healing techniques. Fortunately, the West is finally becoming more aware, and these techniques are now being explored and used.

The Chinese medical 'philosophies' are of vital importance in this particular approach to reflexology. It is my opinion that reflexology evolved in China at the same time as acupuncture and was intended to be utilized in accordance with these concepts. Viewed in this context it is obvious why the Chinese approach to 'dis-ease', incorporating ch'i energy, the meridian system and the elements, is a necessary inclusion.

Some innovative twentieth-century scientists have conducted fascinating research into energy, the human body and the healing process. The work of Dr Harold Saxton Burr, Dr Robert Becker, Dr Bjorn Nordenstrom and Dr Randolph Stone brought energy into modern medicine. Their work should help convince sceptics and encourage more acceptance of energy in healing.

Reflexology is a holistic healing art – a form of therapeutic foot massage – which falls into the realm of 'alternative' medicine. As with most practices in this category, disease is approached from the understanding of man as a complex organism comprised of body, mind and spirit. The object of holistic treatment is to induce a state of balance and harmony throughout the entire organism.

The term 'alternative' medicine in the modern context refers to any form of medicine which does not fall into the mainstream of orthodox Western medicine. This is in fact misrepresentation. Orthodox medicine should be referred to as the 'alternative' due to its relative infancy in the history of medicine. The term 'complementary' is more accurate.

Many practices considered 'alternative' hail from antiquity and are based on traditional folk medicine that existed in all cultures. Every culture and country had its traditional medical system. In those times medicine was a blend of art and science with a generous sprinkling of magic, myth and superstition. As 'modern' medicine evolved, science took precedence and medicine became mechanical, looking at life as a purely chemical phenomenon. Man came to be regarded as a machine made up of a complex collection of parts. Natural medical practices were pushed into the background and suppressed. Most people chose and, to a certain extent, were coerced into believing that modern, more expensive medicine had to be a better form of treatment.

Some decades down the line, the tables are turning. Disillusionment with modern medicine has resulted in a resurgence of interest in, and demand for, safer, more natural forms of therapy. Both orthodox and complementary practices have their place in health care and should ideally work together, as no one therapy can claim to be able to deal with every disease. And neither could claim to be total health care systems. No-one can deny the benefits of modern technology, but in the race for better and more expensive treatment a vital aspect of healing – the human element – has been forced into the background.

WHAT PRICE MODERN MEDICINE?

Said Dr Robert O. Becker: 'The philosophical result of chemical medicine's success has been the belief in the Technological Fix. Drugs became the best or only valid treatment for all ailments.

Prevention, nutrition, exercise, lifestyle, the patient's physical and mental uniqueness, environmental pollutants – all were glossed over. Even today, after so many years and millions of dollars spent for negligible results, it's still assumed that the cure for cancer will be a chemical that kills malignant cells without harming healthy ones. As surgeons become more adept at repairing bodily structures or replacing them with artificial parts, the technological faith came to include the idea that a transplanted kidney, a plastic heart valve or a stainless-steel-and-Teflon hip joint was just as good as the original – or even better because it wouldn't wear out. If a human is merely a chemical machine, then the ultimate human is a robot.'[1]

An apt statement that succinctly expresses the limitations of modern medicine. Man is far more than a collection of working parts. He is a highly sophisticated organism imbued with the vital dimensions of body, mind and spirit. Modern doctors are not always trained to recognize problems beyond the physical. Most complementary therapies recognize that physical imbalance seldom occurs in isolation. Imbalance in mental and spiritual spheres cannot be separated from the physical, so intricately are these interwoven. Disillusionment with orthodox medicine has come about largely due to the fact that many people see it failing in chronic conditions and witness the destructive and disturbing side-effects of drugs and surgery.

Illness is big business. Consumption of drugs in 'civilized' Western countries is astounding. In Britain the pharmaceutical industry turns over £2000 million a year. Unfortunately the public do not reap the benefits – the drug companies do. Pharmacies and drug stores in the Western world overflow with an amazing variety of remedies designed to treat all ills – analgesics, antacids, cough, cold and flu remedies to mention but a few. The fact that no-one has yet discovered a cure for the common cold has not deterred drug companies from flooding the market with an impressive selection of 'suppressors'.

Most modern drugs are manufactured from inorganic chemicals developed in laboratories. Man is an organic organism with a physiology designed to assimilate organic substances, not man-made chemicals. Constant ingestion of drugs can eventually only result in negative conditions as toxic residues accumulate. Almost every drug developed has some destructive side-effect on another function of the body. Drugs suppress disease, relieve symptoms and ease pain but they do not deal with the underlying cause of the 'dis-ease' and eradicate that.

The fact that most of these drugs are tested on animals is also rather disturbing. Apart from the suffering involved, animals are barely an acceptable substitute for the more complex physiology and psychology of *Homo sapiens*. The pitfalls of this practice are evident; few have forgotten the thalidomide scandal. The side-effects of some of the drugs inflicted on the public for decades are only now becoming apparent.

Overexposure to drugs has produced a new kind of disease – iatrogenic disease – illness which is the result of medical or surgical treatment. Exact figures for iatrogenic disease are difficult to assess. Many people do eventually require hospital treatment for this affliction, but there are thousands of victims who battle on through daily life feeling 'not quite right', unaware of the root cause of their malaise.

Many doctors themselves do not understand how some of the orthodox medical treatments work, but continue using them on millions of people. What happened to the maxim *Nil nocere* (First do no harm)? It would be naive to assume this still applies. How many scientists, chemists and doctors test the drugs they develop and prescribe on themselves before prescribing them to the public?

Look at the most commonly used and easily available product on the market – aspirin. Until recently no-one knew how aspirin worked yet for over seventy years it has been the most widely used medicine in the world. It may be most effective in treating mild pain and headaches, but long-term use can be destructive. The active ingredient in aspirin – acetylsalicylic acid – is a substance for which the human body has no use. Continual use of aspirin can increase the risk of stomach ulcers and kidney disease, block the uptake of Vitamin C and lower folic acid levels.[2]

Cortisone – another modern-day wonder-drug – is also potentially dangerous. Today it is used to treat over a hundred different ailments including cancer, arthritis, kidney disease, hay-fever and allergies. In America, 29 million prescriptions for cortisone are written every year. Cortisone doesn't cure, it suppresses, and prolonged use can cause the body to stop producing its own cortisone.[3]

Yet another unfortunate oversight in the field of orthodox medicine is the lack of emphasis on nutrition. Considering that the human body is constructed from the food we eat, it would seem necessary to include nutrition as an integral aspect of medical training. This is not the case. Nutrition does not feature on the medical training curriculum.

Modern medicine is also rapidly becoming elitist. The cost of health care is escalating at such a rate that few people can afford adequate medical care. And health care systems will deteriorate as governments find it increasingly difficult to subsidize the exorbitant costs.

There can be no doubt that modern medicine has contributed greatly to the improvement of health care. For example, prior to the advent of penicillin, disease epidemics were devastating. Numerous diseases which once had high mortality rates can now be easily controlled with penicillin.

Surgery is another wonder of modern medicine, a miracle of modern technology that provides impressive and life-saving treatment for numerous conditions. Unfortunately, relatively little surgery performed today falls into the life-saving category. Many operations – tonsillectomies, appendectomies, hysterectomies, gall bladder removal and hernias – deal with symptoms resulting from self-abuse and could probably have been prevented with correct nutrition and lifestyle.

As the object of both orthodox and complementary medicine is to cure disease and be of assistance to the human race, the most positive prognosis would be that both recognize their place in health care and work together for the benefit of all. The best complementary therapies combined with the finest in technological medicine would be a great breakthrough in health care. To quote a World Health Organisation Report: 'For too long traditional systems of medicine and 'modern' medicine have gone their separate ways in mutual antipathy. Yet are not their goals identical – to improve the health of mankind and thereby the quality of life? Only the blinkered mind would assume that each has nothing to do with the other.'[4]

A QUESTION OF ENERGY

As the concept of energy in healing is an important facet of this book, a short introduction is necessary to justify this and illustrate that energy is the core which links all living things in the universe.

All matter is made up of energy. The holistic health philosophy considers the human body as a dynamic energy system in a constant state of change. We are all an expression of energy and this energy permeates all living organisms. Because we cannot perceive energy with the naked eye, we find it difficult to comprehend. This does not mean it does not exist.

In Chinese and Ayurvedic medicine, health is seen as the fluent and harmonious movement of energies at subtle levels. In the East these energies have various names. The Indian yogis call it *prana*; to the Tibetan lamas it is *lung-gom*. It is known as *sakia-tundra* or *ki* to the Japanese Shinto, and the Chinese call it *ch'i*. In the West it is loosely translated at 'vital energy', 'vital force' or 'life-force'.

Ch'i is difficult to define. A good description is the following passage from *The Secret of the Golden Flower: A Chinese Book of Life*: 'Heaven created water through One. This is the true energy of the great One. If man attains the One he becomes alive; if he loses it he dies. But even if man lives in the energy (vital breath) he does not see the energy, just as fishes live in water but do not see the water. Man dies when he has not vital breath, just as fishes perish when deprived of water. If one guards this true energy, one can prolong the span of life and can apply the method of creating an immortal body.'[5]

Vital energy represents some form of electricity. This does not mean it *is* electricity, but that its behaviour, responses and reactions indicate that many of the laws applying to electricity also apply to vital energy. Every life function depends on this energy. According to Far Eastern tradition it circulates in the viscera, the flesh and ultimately permeates every living cell and tissue. This energy is considered as having clearly distinct and established pathways, definite direction of flow, and characteristic behaviour as well-defined as any other circulation such as blood and the vascular system.[6]

A great deal of research into ch'i and meridians has been conducted in the last few decades, but access to this research is limited for Westerners, as it is published in Chinese. Apparently, Chinese scientists are piecing together the fundamental characteristics of life energy. So far, they know it has four characteristics: electric, magnetic, infra-red and infrasonic. So many scientists in China are now concentrating their work on ch'i that a special branch of science – chiconology – has developed. Says Dr Joshua Le,

consultant to the British College of Acupuncture in London: 'Many scientists now believe the electromagnetic recordings of ch'i have proved its existence. Everyone has ch'i, so it should be acknowledged by everyone, even GPs in the Western world. It's as real as any blood vessels. The significance of this acceptance in medicine worldwide could be tremendous.'[7]

The movement of energy is based on or due to a relationship which sets up two opposing fields; a 'polarity'. In Chinese philosophy this polarity relationship is called 'yin and yang'. Says Ted Kaptchuk in his book *The Web That Has No Weaver*: 'Yin-yang theory is based on the philosophical construct of two polar complements, called yin and yang. These complementary opposites are neither forces nor material entities. Nor are they mythical concepts that transcend rationality. Rather, they are convenient labels used to describe how things function in relation to each other and to the universe. They are used to explain the continuous process of natural change. But yin and yang are not only a set of correspondences; they also represent a way of thinking. In this system of thought all things are seen as parts of a whole. No entity can ever be isolated from its relationship to other entities; no thing can exist in and of itself. There are no absolutes. Yin and yang must contain within themselves the possibility of opposition and change.'[8]

In physical terms man can be reduced to a collection of electromagnetic fields. What we perceive as solid tissue is actually a mass of cells made up of chemical substances which are collections of atoms. Every atom carries an electrical charge. An atom consists of protons (positively charged), neutrons (no charge) and electrons (negatively charged). Electrons are more easily dislodged from atoms than protons so are the main carriers of electric charge.[9] Thus, at the atomic level the body is a mass of energy fields all influencing each other.

The first 'modern' scientific evidence of energy and the human body came from Dr Harold Saxton Burr, Professor of Anatomy at Yale in the 1930s. He was convinced of the existence of 'animal electricity' and developed apparatus to measure electrical potential even in very small organisms. He proved that man, plants and animals are surrounded by a life-field (L-field). Each produces an electric field that can be measured some distance away from the body and which mirrors and could possibly even control changes in that body. 'Animals and plants,' said Burr, 'are essentially electric and show a change in voltage gradient associated with fundamental biological activity.'[10]

Burr, the Editor of the *Yale Journal of Biology and Medicine*, published twenty-eight papers outlining the bio-electric nature of menstruation, ovulation, sleep, growth, healing and disease. Burr and his colleagues observed that changes in life-fields indicated changes taking place in the organisms producing these fields and used these to chart the course of health, predict illness, follow progress of healing in a wound, pinpoint movement of ovulation, diagnose psychic trauma and measure the depth of hypnosis.[11] This energy field or 'aura' can be perceived by 'sensitive' people, and has been 'proven' to exist by Kirlian photography – a technique which photographs the aura.

Another Western physician who made an invaluable contribution to the use of electric energy in healing is Dr Robert O. Becker. An orthopaedic surgeon, he was interested in the possibility of electric current regenerating broken bones. After many experiments involving salamanders and frogs to examine electric currents at the site of injury, Becker proved the efficacy of his theory. Now patients can have small hearing aid batteries that produce a sustained negative charge implanted close to severe fractures that are reluctant to heal – with dramatic results. He was also interested in electricity as a factor in the overall control of cell differentiation and growth and proved that the right kind of current could inhibit infection, relieve pain, halt osteomyelitis, restore muscle control, repair intestinal ruptures, close holes in the heart, regenerate nerve cords and replace lost parts in the brain.[12]

Further research conducted by Dr Bjorn Nordenstrom was revealed in the American magazine *Discover*. The headline read: 'Electric Man. Dr Bjorn Nordenstrom claims to have found in the human body a heretofore unknown universe of electrical activity that's the very foundation of the healing process and is as critical to well-being as the flow of blood. If he's right he has made the most profound biochemical discovery of the century.' Inside, a thirteen-page article detailed Nordenstrom's discovery of electrical polarities in the bloodstream and how he is manipulating the natural electrical circuits he has found to disperse tumours.[13]

Dr Randolph Stone, who died in 1981 in India at the age of ninety-one, combined Eastern and Western understanding to develop Polarity Therapy. A qualified osteopath and chiropractor, he came to define techniques for balancing the energy flow in human beings through his knowledge of Eastern wisdom, his understanding of the inner structure of the universe and of the *gunas* described in Hindu literature. He developed, practised and taught Polarity Therapy in California and India with great success.[14]

The West has finally discovered what the East has acknowledged for thousands of years – that electrical energy forms the basis of all life. More people are beginning to accept that the physical world is part of a much larger whole – a whole that, unfortunately, most of us cannot physically perceive. We pick up only a tiny fraction of what is really going on around us, because our concepts of life are limited by our five physical senses. To quote Lyall Watson from his book

Supernature II: 'Earth and everything in it is under constant bombardment. We are battered by a ceaseless barrage of more than a hundred million impulses every second . . . a confusing avalanche of raw knowledge with which we cannot hope to deal.

'The flood ranges from highly energetic cosmic rays, whose origin remains mysterious, but which at all latitudes have the intriguing property of coming rushing in largely from the west, through shortwave gamma and X-radiation, which passes with relative ease through our bodies; to ultraviolet and infra-red light waves that leave us with Vitamin D and radiant heat; and a wide band of radio frequencies that bring us sound broadcasting, television, radar and a scattering of information about distant galaxies in collision.

'Most of this news is irrelevant. It contributes nothing to an organism battling for survival on a much more limited field. To prevent being overwhelmed by the flood, we have evolved barriers which filter out the stuff we don't need.

'So, from all the pyrotechnics of electromagnetism our senses select just that narrow band of radiation that represents the visible spectrum – those wavelengths which lie between 375 and 775 billionths of a metre. We look on the world through a tiny slit, and this narrow window on reality is even further restricted by the censorship taking place between the eye and the brain.'[15]

The human ear responds to sounds within a frequency range of approximately 30–16,000 cycles per second. Human vision responds to wavelengths from 380 to 760 millimicrons. Of approximately fifty octaves of electromagnetic radiations, our eyes pick up less than one.

From the barrage of electromagnetic waves in the environment living organisms select only those necessary for their survival. Although our brains are not geared to pick up TV waves, radio waves and ultrasonic frequencies, we do not doubt their existence, so how can we doubt the existence of electrical energy in the body merely because we can't see it?

All life on earth is intricately interwoven with the natural rhythms and laws of the universe. Every organism regulates its metabolic activity in cycles attuned to the fluctuations of the earth, sun and moon. So we humans are directly and indirectly affected by various cosmic forces beyond our control. To quote Lyall Watson again: 'Our internal clocks are clearly tied to the rhythms provided by the planet and its nearest neighbours in the solar system. We wake and sleep, sweat and shiver, urinate and respirate in time with cosmic cues that are often so subtle that medical science has had a hard time taking them seriously. But an avalanche of studies in the last (few) decades on insomnia, menstrual irregularity and stress in those suffering from cyclic disturbances such as jet lag, has turned the tide. It is now more widely accepted that functional integrity, the basic processes of growth and control, and the efficient working of the central nervous system are all maintained to a very large extent by our electromagnetic environment.'[16]

This brief synopsis barely encompasses the vastness of phenomena occurring around us all the time, but is intended to emphasize the importance of the interconnectedness of all things and how health is dependent on vital 'electric' forces. The optimum state for each individual is to live in harmony with nature and the surrounding environment. And it is the role of the reflexologist, working in accordance with the holistic philosophy, to help people to work towards and achieve this state of balance.

History

*How beautiful upon the mountains are the feet of him
that bringeth good tidings, that publisheth peace.*

ISAIAH 3:7

FEET FACTS

Feet have an illustrious and intriguing history. People often view their feet as an alien part of their anatomy, seldom considering the important role of these pedal appendages, but anthropologists regard the foot as the definitive human physical trait. When the first anthropoid straightened up from a four-legged crouch approximately fifty million years ago, a chain of events was set in motion. These adaptive measures are considered highly significant in the history of evolution.

The feet, originally designed to carry one-quarter of the body weight each, had to adjust to carrying half each. The spinal column, originally an arch between forefeet and back feet, had to adapt to the upright position. With these modifications, blood circulation altered, as well as the mechanics of breathing, the placement of our internal organs and our outlook on life. The thumblike big toe moved into the same plane as the other toes, and the heel dropped to rest on the ground to support the body weight more efficiently. The arches evolved to contribute to our stride. Locomotive processes transferred to lower extremities leaving the rest of the body free to perform other tasks.[1]

In bygone times, feet were held in high regard. Leonardo da Vinci called the foot 'a masterpiece of engineering and a work of art'. He was not wrong. Considering the size of the feet in relation to the body they support, the humble feet are nothing short of remarkable.

Fascination with the foot dates way back and references appear in mythology, religion and culture. The best-known mythological reference is Achilles' heel. The story goes that while dipping Achilles in waters to render him invulnerable, his mother held him by one heel. This small part of his anatomy that missed submersion was ultimately the cause of his demise. He died in the Trojan War when a poisoned arrow pierced this overlooked heel. The term 'Achilles' heel' is still used today to refer to a weak spot.[2]

The Greek foot – a term derived from ancient mythology – originally referred to goddesses with longer second toes which was symbolic of their male powers.[3] And virgin goddesses were always depicted covering their feet to protect their chastity as feet were considered extremely private parts. Revealing the feet was perceived as the equivalent of a blatant proposition.[4]

Eminent authors and poets – from Shakespeare and Tennyson to Oscar Wilde – praised the feet in their works. And feet often arise in religious customs. The mention of feet as metaphor is often quoted in the Bible – specifically in the instance of Christ washing the feet of his disciples at the Last Supper. The Asian custom of foot kissing was a gesture of submission towards a person of lofty status like a pope or a saint. The removal of shoes at the threshold of holy places is observed by Buddhists, Hindus and Muslims. This, too, appears in the Bible – when God said to Moses: 'Put off thy shoes from thy feet, for the place whereon thou standest is holy ground.'[5]

In Chinese cultures, a woman's foot was regarded as the ultimate sex symbol. To render the feet the most attractive parts of the anatomy and mould them into the desired shape, women's feet were bound. This prevented bones developing in the usual way and stunted foot growth. This uncomfortable and unkind practice has fortunately been discontinued.[6]

The foot is a finely tuned mechanical masterpiece which has lost some ground in the popularity stakes over the years. But with increased interest in holistic healing practices comes the realization that feet play a fundamental role in health and well-being.

THE ROOTS OF REFLEXOLOGY

The roots of reflexology are embedded way back in ancient history when pressure therapies were recognized as preventive and therapeutic medicine. Exactly where and how it all began is somewhat elusive, but evidence indicates that therapeutic foot massage has been practised throughout history by a variety of cultures.

Ancient History

A widely held theory is that reflexology originated in China some 5000 years ago. Many reputable reflexologists have stated their belief in this theory even though concrete proof is evasive. Egyptian and Babylonian cultures developed before Chinese culture, however, and Egypt

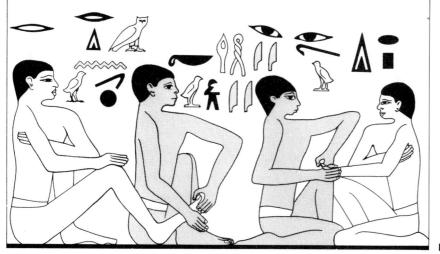

Fig.1

contributed a valuable piece of historical evidence.

The oldest documentation depicting the practice of reflexology was unearthed in Egypt. This evidence, a pictograph dated around 2500–2330 BC, was found in the tomb of an Egyptian physician, Ankmahor, at Saqqara. According to evidence found in the tomb, Ankmahor was a most influential person – second only to the king.

The scene in the pictograph in figure 1 depicts two darker-skinned men working on the feet and hands of two men with lighter skin. In ancient Egypt, advanced civilizations and knowledge came from the south where the darker skin was prized. One explanation of the pictograph comes from the Egyptian Mohamed el Awany: 'The dark people with the hair in the curly African style are from upper Egypt and are obviously the practitioners, who have come from the south to treat those from Lower Egypt who have lighter coloured bodies and straight hair. The positions of the patients is different. The patient on the left has his right hand on his right knee and his left hand under his right armpit. The other patient is the opposite. There is a relationship between the kind of problem the patient has and where the practitioner touches. This determines the points of pressure he and the patient use. In this case, the patient is touching the reflex point under his arm where he feels the corresponding pain.' According to the Papyrus Institute in Cairo the hieroglyphics above the scene read: 'Do not let it be painful,' says one of the patients. 'I do as you please,' an attendant replies.[7]

Another theory claims that a form of reflex therapy was passed down to the American Indians by the Incas. Again, no specific evidence supports this theory. However, the use of reflex pressure applied to the feet as a healing therapy has been practised by the North American Indians for generations. For centuries the Cherokee Indians of North Carolina have acknowledged the importance of feet in maintaining physical, mental and spiritual balance. The Bear Clan from this tribe who live in the back hills of the Allehjanies can attest to this.

Jenny Wallace, a Cherokee Indian from the Bear Clan, practises as a foot therapist in America today. In the tribe, she is known as a 'moon-maiden' – a title bestowed on a person who, as a young girl, exhibits natural intuitive healing talents, and is chosen by the tribe to develop this talent further. According to her: 'In my tribe working on the feet is a very important healing art and is part of a sacred ceremony that you don't have to be ill to take part in. The feet walk upon the earth and through this your spirit is connected to the universe. Our feet are our contact with the earth and the energies that flow through it.'[8]

This knowledge of foot reflex therapy may have been lost to antiquity had it not been for enquiring medical minds of the late nineteenth and early twentieth centuries. People intrigued by the concept of reflex therapy instigated a resurgence of interest in the study of reflexes. The study and development of reflex therapy by pioneering Europeans and enterprising Americans laid the foundations of reflexology as we know it today.

THE DEVELOPMENT OF ZONE THERAPY – THE FOUNDATION OF MODERN REFLEXOLOGY

The European Influence

In Europe a form of reflexology was known and practised as far back as the fourteenth century. According to Harry Bond Bressler in his book *Zone Therapy*, 'Pressure therapy was well known in the middle countries of Europe and was practised by the working classes of those countries as well as by those who catered to the diseases of royalty and the upper classes. Dr Adamus and Dr A'tatis wrote a book on the subject of zone therapy which was published in 1582. In Leipzig Dr Ball wrote another book on the same subject, and it was published soon after the other book.'[9]

The scientific basis of reflex study had its roots in neurological studies conducted in the 1890s by Sir Henry Head of London. In 1898 he discovered zones on the skin which became hypersensitive to pressure when an organ connected by nerves to this skin region was diseased. After years of clinical research Head established what became known as 'Head's Zones' or 'zones of hyperalgesia'.

Russian work on reflexes began from a psychological point of view. The founder of Russian physiology, Ivan Sechenov (who discovered the cerebral inhibition of spinal reflexes), published a paper in 1870 titled 'Who Must Investigate the Problems of Psychology and How?'. Psychologists under Vladimir Bekhterev, who founded Leningrad's Brain Institute, picked up the challenge and studied it through reflexes. At the same time Ivan Pavlov (1849–1936) read Sechenov's work and acknowledged that his book *Reflexes of the Brain* was the most important theoretical inspiration for his own work on conditioning. Pavlov took Sechenov's theoretical outline and submitted it to methodical experimental study. Through this, Pavlov developed the theory of conditioned reflexes — namely that there is a simple and direct relationship between a stimulus and a response. Pavlov found that practically any stimulus can act as a conditioning stimulus to produce a conditioned response.[10]

Today the Russians continue to pursue the study of reflexology both from the physiological and psychological point of view. They have scientifically tested the effect of reflex therapy on patients with a variety of problems and have found reflexology to be an effective complement to traditional medicine.[11]

At the same time, the Germans were also looking into the treatment of disease by massage. In the late 1890s and early 1900s massage techniques developed in Germany became known as 'reflex massage'. This was the first time that the benefits of massage techniques were credited to reflex actions.

Apparently Dr Alfons Cornelius was possibly the first to apply massage to 'reflex zones'. The story goes that in 1893, Cornelius suffered from an infection. In the course of his convalescence he received a daily massage. At the spa he noticed how effective the massages of one particular medical officer were. This man worked longer on areas he found painful. This concept inspired Cornelius. After examining himself, Cornelius instructed his masseur to work only on the painful areas. His pain quickly disappeared and in four weeks he completely recovered. This led him to pursue the use of pressure in his own medical practice. He published his manuscript 'Druckpunkte' or 'Pressure Points, The Origin and Significance' in 1902.[12]

Europeans went on to expand on the research initiated by the above-mentioned people. But credit for putting modern reflexology on the map must go to the Americans.

The American Influence

Dr William Fitzgerald, commonly known as the founder of Zone Therapy, was born in Connecticut, USA, in 1872. He graduated in medicine from the University of Vermont in 1895 and practised in hospitals in Vienna and London.

In Vienna he came into contact with the work of Dr H. Bressler who had been investigating the possibility of treating organs with pressure points. Fitzgerald continued his research while Head Physician at the Hospital for Diseases of the Ear, Nose and Throat in Hartford, Connecticut, testing out many of his theories on his patients. Through knowledge he gained in

Europe and his own research, Fitzgerald found that if pressure was applied on the fingers, it would create a local anaesthetic effect on the hand, arm and shoulder, right up to the jaw, face, ear and nose. He applied pressure using tight bands of elastic on the middle section of each finger or small clamps which he placed on the tips. He was able to carry out minor surgical operations just using this pressure technique.[13]

Dr Fitzgerald divided the body into zones, which he used for his anaesthetic effect. By exerting pressure on a specific part of the body he learned to predict which other parts of the body would be affected. Fitzgerald established ten equal longitudinal zones running the length of the body from the top of the head to the tips of the toes. The number ten corresponds to the fingers and toes and therefore provides a simple numbering system. Each finger and toe falls into one zone. Imagine a line drawn through the centre of the body with five zones on either side of this line. The thumb and big toe fall into zone one and the small finger and toe both fall into zone five. The zones are of equal width and extend right through the body from front to back. The theory is that parts of the body found within a certain zone will be linked with one another by the energy flow within the zone and can therefore affect one another.

In his book *Zone Therapy* Fitzgerald describes how he came upon the concept of zone therapy: 'I accidentally discovered that pressure with a cotton-tipped probe on the mucocutaneous margin (where the skin joins the mucous membrane) of the nose gave an anaesthetic result as though a cocaine solution had been applied. I further found that there were many spots in the nose, mouth, throat, and on both surfaces of the tongue which, when pressed firmly, deadened definite areas of sensation. Also, that pressures exerted over any body eminence, on the hands, feet, or over the joints, produced the same characteristic results in pain relief. I found also

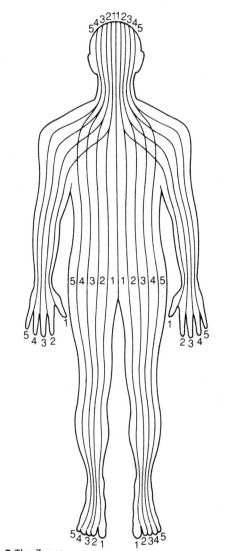

Fig. 2 The Zones

that when pain was relieved, the condition that produced the pain was most generally relieved. This led to my 'mapping out' these various areas and their associated connections, and also to noting the conditions influenced through them. This science I have named zone therapy.'[14]

Fitzgerald and colleague Dr Edwin Bowers were so enthusiastic about their discoveries that they developed a unique method for convincing their colleagues about the validity of the zone theory. They would apply pressure to the sceptic's hand then stick a pin in the area of the face anaesthetized by the pressure. Such dramatic proof made believers of those who witnessed it. In 1915, Bowers wrote the article that first publicly described this treatment and called it 'zone therapy'. This was published in *Everybody's Magazine* and entitled 'To Stop That Toothache Squeeze Your Toe!'[15]

This of course elicited much interest and controversy, and Fitzgerald was often called on to publicly prove the validity of his theories. One such incident was reported in a newspaper on 29 April 1934, under the headline 'Mystery of Zone Therapy Explained'. The article tells of a dinner party at which one of the guests was Fitzgerald, and another a well-known concert singer who had announced that the upper register tones of her voice had gone flat. The article noted that throat specialists had been unable to discover the cause of this affliction. Dr Fitzgerald, according to the article, asked to examine the fingers and toes of the singer. After his examination he told her that the cause of the loss of her upper tones was a callus on her right big toe. After applying pressure to the corresponding part in the same zone for a few minutes, the patient remarked that the pain in her toe had disappeared. Then, to quote from the article: 'the doctor asked her to try the tone of the upper register. Miraculously, it would seem to us, the singer reached two tones higher than she had ever done before.'[16]

In 1917, the combined work of Dr Fitzgerald and Dr Bowers was published in the book *Zone Therapy*. Diagrams of the zones of the feet and the corresponding division of the ten zones of the body appeared in the first edition of this book. But the reflex zones of the feet, so crucial to modern reflexology, were not singled out for any special attention by Fitzgerald.

Fitzgerald and his theories were not enthusiastically received by the medical profession.

One physician did believe in his work – Dr Joseph Shelby Riley. Fitzgerald taught zone therapy to Riley and his wife, Elizabeth, and they used this method in their practice for many years. Riley refined the techniques and made the first detailed diagrams and drawings of the reflex points located in the feet. He added to Fitzgerald's longitudinal zones his discovery of eight horizontal divisions which also govern the body. His first book *Zone Therapy Simplified* was published in 1919. He wrote four books in which large portions were devoted to zone therapy.[17]

Fitzgerald, Bower and Riley developed and refined the theory of zone therapy, but it was Riley's assistant Eunice Ingham who probably made the greatest contribution to the establishment of modern reflexology. It was through her untiring research and dedication that reflexology finally came into its own. She separated the work on the reflexes of the feet from zone therapy in general.

Eunice Ingham (1879–1974) should be called the Mother of Modern Reflexology. She used zone therapy in her work but felt that the feet should be specific targets for therapy because of their highly sensitive nature. She charted the feet in relation to the zones and their effects on the rest of the anatomy until she had evolved on the feet themselves a 'map' of the entire body. So successful was her work that her reputation spread and she is now recognized as the founder of foot reflexology.

Her nephew Dwight Byers was often guinea pig for his aunt's research. He recalls: 'My earliest recollection of my aunt's work was in 1935 when, during the summer, she lived at Conesus Lake, one of the Finger Lakes in upper New York State. She expanded her research by giving treatments to the residents of this small village. I particularly remember those treatments that year because it was the first time I ever found relief from my annual bouts with asthma and hay fever. She would eagerly practise her theories on my feet while explaining the reflex theory as she worked. I must confess that, to a youth who was wheezing and sneezing, theory took second place to what blessed relief she was able to give me. Interestingly enough, it was while treating me that she convinced herself that in less serious cases, only a few treatments a week sufficed to help most patients.'[18]

Eunice Ingham took her work to the public and the non-medical community because she realized that lay people could learn the proper reflexology techniques to help themselves, their families and friends. She was called on to speak at conventions and shared her knowledge with chiropodists, massage practitioners and physiotherapists, naturopaths and osteopaths. She travelled throughout America for over thirty years as she taught her method through books, charts and seminars to thousands of people in and out of the medical profession. She wrote two books, *Stories The Feet Can Tell* (1938) and *Stories The Feet Have Told* (1963). Today her legacy continues under the direction of her nephew Dwight Byers who runs the International Institute of Reflexology in St Petersburg.[19]

Zone theory is considered the basis of modern foot reflexology and most reflexologists use zone therapy as a useful adjunct to their work. However, the time has come to take foot reflexology a step further and expand on existing knowledge by combining it with the ancient Chinese system of meridian therapy. Many believe foot reflexology had its origins in China and developed around the same time as acupuncture. Despite the fact that no definite links can be made, a combination of what is now regarded as primarily a Western development with an ancient Eastern treatment can only be beneficial.

THE CHINESE CONNECTION

There can be little doubt that a strong link exists between reflexology and acupuncture. They are certainly based on similar ideas. Both are considered meridian therapies as they propose that energy lines link the hands and feet to various body parts. This enables the whole body to be treated by working on the reflex areas. Acupuncture went from strength to strength in the East but reflexology was, for some unknown reason, lost and forgotten until its recent re-emergence in the West.

The Chinese had divided the body into longitudinal meridians by approximately 2500 BC whereas the similar idea of zones came to Western awareness as late as the 1900s, as we have seen. Acupuncture, despite its popularity in the East, was an unknown art in the West until 1883 when Dutch physician Ten Thyne wrote a treatise on the subject.

Reflexology definitely has some relationship with acupuncture, shiatsu and acupressure. According to acupuncture, the body has twelve pairs of meridians as well as two special meridians known as vessels. Together these constitute the body's energy system which works to maintain the health of the organism. These meridians are pathways through which the energy of the universe circulates throughout the body organs and keeps the universe and the body in harmony. The acupuncturist believes that illness or pain occurs when the pathways become blocked, disrupting the energy flow and breaking the body's harmony. The Chinese, in acupuncture, developed the use of needles to unblock these pathways. In shiatsu, the Japanese use direct thumb and finger pressure on acupuncture meridian points to achieve similar results.[20] Reflexologists also work on acupuncture and acupressure points but only those found in the feet. Through increased awareness of meridians one can practise reflexology more effectively as meridians provide profound insight into the disease pathway, and are therefore a most useful diagnostic tool.

The Chinese were undoubtedly aware of the

importance of the feet in treating disease. In AD 1017 Dr Wang Wei had a human figure cast in bronze on which were marked those points on the body important for acupuncture. When this knowledge was put into practice in treating the sick, practitioners positioned the needles in the appropriate areas of the body and then applied deep pressure therapy on the soles of the inside and outside edge of both feet. They then applied a concentrated pressure on the big toe. The reason they used the feet in conjunction with the acupuncture needles was to channel extra energy through the body. Dr Wei said that the feet were the most sensitive part of all and contained great energizing areas.[21]

As more evidence becomes available one can barely refute the fact that, although not visible to the naked eye, energy pathways do exist. Russian physiologists have carried out extensive studies using encephalography, electrocardiography and X-rays. These studies, which involve measuring the electrical potential of the skin at the classical acupuncture points, have verified basic claims for acupuncture and related its effects to reflex action.

To date, most reflexologists have worked with the theory of energy zones described by Dr Fitzgerald. Although this theory has stood reflexology in good stead and contributed greatly to the development of the modern therapy, I personally do not adhere to it. I believe the effects elicited by massaging the feet are largely the result of stimulating the six main meridians that run through the feet. Fitzgerald recognized an energy connection between the feet and other parts of the body and without his pioneering work reflexology would not be where it is today. But as the Eastern concept of the meridian system was unknown in the West at the time of his research, the connection with the meridians was not recognized. I, however, am convinced that the energy channels linking the feet to other organs and body parts are the meridians described in Chinese medicine.

It is not the object of the book to prove that reflexology is directly related to meridians. The object is to illustrate that a combination of knowledge – modern reflexology techniques and the Eastern meridian system – can be of enormous benefit to patient and practitioner. As acupuncture and reflexology are concerned with balancing energy flow in order to stimulate the body's own healing potential and restore a state of health, and both are concerned with treating illness in a holistic manner, it seems logical to combine reflexology with meridian therapy in order to provide a more comprehensive and effective treatment programme.

CHAPTER TWO

What is Reflexology and How Does it Work?

*For her feet have touched the meadows
And left the daisies rosy.*
ALFRED, LORD TENNYSON

Reflexology is a gentle art, a fascinating science and an extremely effective form of therapeutic foot massage that has carved an impressive niche in the field of complementary medicine. It is a science because it is based on physiological and neurological study; and an art because much depends on how skilfully the practitioner applies his or her knowledge, and the dynamics which occur between practitioner and recipient.[1]

Reflexology is a holistic healing technique – the term 'holistic' derived from the Greek word *holos* which means 'whole' – and as such aims to treat the individual as an entity incorporating body, mind and spirit. Reflexologists do not isolate a disease and treat it symptomatically, nor do they work specifically on a problem organ or system, but on the whole person with the object of inducing a state of balance and harmony. The art of reflex foot massage must not be confused with basic foot massage or body massage in general. It is a specific pressure technique which works on precise reflex points on the feet, based on the premise that reflex areas on the feet

correspond with all body parts. As the feet represent a microcosm of the body, all organs, glands and other body parts are laid out in a similar arrangement on the feet.

The phenomenon of microcosmic representation of body parts in different areas of the body is also evident in the iris of the eye, the ear and the hands. The corresponding areas on the feet are, however, easier to locate as they cover a larger area and are more specific, rendering them easier to work on. Pressure is applied to the reflex areas using specific thumb and finger techniques. This causes physiological changes to take place in the body as the body's own healing potential is stimulated. Thus, the feet can play a major role in attaining and maintaining better health.

The simplicity of reflexology treatment belies its efficacy. No high-tech, complicated equipment is necessary. The technique is so simple it does not require years of training to master. A good practitioner needs a sensitive but sturdy pair of hands, a genuine desire to ease pain and suffering, compassion, intuition and an understanding of human nature. The relationship between the recipient and practitioner is an important aspect of the healing process. The practitioner acts as mediator to activate the client's healing potential.

The goal of reflexology is to trigger the return to homeostasis – a state of equilibrium or balance. The most important step towards achieving this is to reduce tension and induce relaxation. To quote Kevin and Barbara Kunz from their book *The Complete Guide to Foot Reflexology*: 'If reflexology never accomplished anything more than combatting stress with relaxation, it is serving its purpose very well.'[2]

Relaxation is the first step to normalization. When the body is relaxed healing is possible. Professional massage of the reflexes of the feet will establish which parts of the body are out of balance and therefore not working efficiently. Treatment can then be given to correct these imbalances and return the body to an optimum state of health. This form of therapy is useful for treating ill health, and effective in maintaining good health and preventing illness. With foot reflex massage, health problems can be detected early and treatment given to prevent more serious symptoms from developing.

As a holistic therapy, reflexology aims to treat the body as a whole and endeavours to get to the root cause of disease and treat this, not the symptom. For best results, the participation of the client is required. Ultimately the reflexologist is not responsible for the client's health. In all holistic therapies, emphasis is placed on taking responsibility for one's own state of health. In orthodox medicine, the tendency is to hand over responsibility to the doctor and expect him to cure all ills. This is a bit of a tall order.

'Dis-ease' is a direct result of one's own thoughts and actions. The mind is immensely powerful and affects every cell in the body. This causes chemical changes to take place. Negative emotions, like anxiety, grief, fear and worry – widespread in modern society – will cause negative repercussions. 'Why poison the body with poisonous thoughts?' said Eunice Ingham. How right she was. Negative attitudes will never facilitate a cure, but a positive attitude goes a long way towards attaining and sustaining a healthy body and mind.

For the sufferer it is imperative to be willing to let go of disease and take an active role in the treatment. A reflexology practitioner will be compassionate, caring and dedicated to the person's welfare, but no practitioner can decide for someone that he or she is going to get well. The client must take that responsibility. A genuine desire for health and willingness to let go of disease is of vital importance to any healing *process*. People venturing into the field of complementary medicine must understand that there is no such thing as an instant cure – it is a healing process. Most diseases have taken time to manifest and will therefore take time to eradicate. The human body is amazingly resilient. It usually takes an enormous amount of abuse before manifesting signs of disease, and will respond extremely well if treated kindly.

The human body is a magnificent machine. Thousands of parts work together to keep the body functioning at optimum levels. The negative effects of emotions, attitudes, stress, lifestyle and diet can throw the body out of sync, causing malfunctions. If one part ceases to function efficiently, the whole suffers. Then the minor aches and pains and general fatigue that are often forerunners of more serious complaints begin to manifest. The analogy of a car is often used to describe the workings of the body. To get maximum response from your car you have to keep it in good working order. If one part isn't working properly, the whole car suffers and has to go to the garage for a tune-up. Or you trade it in for a new one. Reflexology can be considered the equivalent of a tune-up – a body tune-up.

And as you can't trade your body in for a new one, it makes sense to treat the one you have well.

The reflexologist doesn't heal – only the body heals. But reflexology helps to balance all the body systems, stimulating an underactive area and calming an overactive one. It is harmless to those areas functioning properly. As all body systems are closely interrelated, anything which affects one part will ultimately affect the whole. Numerous practitioners, after years of study and practice, have concluded that reflexology works on a number of levels – physiological, psychological and spiritual.

REFLEXOLOGY REVITALIZES ENERGY AND REBALANCES THE WHOLE SYSTEM

The body is a dynamic energy field. The Chinese discovered that this energy – ch'i, – circulates along twelve meridian pathways within the body. (This aspect is discussed in more depth in Section 4, Chapter 2.) The six main meridians which penetrate the major organs of the body are found in the feet – specifically in the toes. Massaging these helps clear blockages along the meridians and encourages the vital body energy to flow unimpeded.

The theory that some form of energy animates the body is now more widely acknowledged. And the belief that this energy is revitalized through reflexology treatment is expounded by many modern reflexologists. Says Ann Gillanders: 'The body is based on an electrical circuit and like normal circuits has negative and positive poles. Reflexology is a method of contacting the electrical centres in the body and has been used for centuries to create a smooth flow of vibratory energy through the body by contacting various points in the feet which relate to various organs, glands and cells.'[3]

Doreen Bayley, the woman who introduced reflexology to Britain, has this to say: 'There is, I believe, an electrical impulse triggered off by pressure massage on a tender reflex and there is a subtle flow which brings that remarkable return of vitality to the patient even while receiving treatment. I believe that the electrical impulse acts on the body in the same way that the stimulus of light acts on the retina of the eye. It has been proven that the action of the full spectrum of light on the retina of the eye, in which are embedded the endings of the optic nerve, produces an electrical impulse which is carried to the hypothalamus, from whence it passes down to the pituitary gland, which passes down to the lesser glands, thereby activating all the functions of the body. It is my belief that the work upon the reflexes produces similar results.'[4]

And Eunice Ingham states: 'The nerves of our body may be likened to an electrical system. It will be our ability to make normal contact with the electricity in the ground, through our feet and from the elements or atmosphere surrounding us, that will determine the degree of power we are able to manifest in proper functioning of the glands. Trying to get a normal contact when there is congestion in these nerve terminals in the feet is like trying to put a plug into a defective fixture.'[5]

For the human organism to function at optimum capacity, energy must flow unimpeded and the yin and yang energy currents must complement each other. Reflexology opens up the energy pathways, energizing the physical, emotional and mental aspects of the client. The specific techniques for applying pressure to the feet create channels for healing energy to circulate to all parts of the body. When the body is 'out of balance' it is not functioning efficiently. Reflexology helps return the body to a dynamic state of balance.

When the reflexes on the feet are stimulated, an involuntary response is elicited in organs and glands connected by energy pathways to these specific reflexes. A chain reaction is set in motion causing physiological changes to occur throughout all the body systems.

REFLEXOLOGY VERSUS THE STRESS SYNDROME

One of the most important benefits of reflexology is its efficacy in reducing stress. Approximately 70 per cent of disorders can be related to stress and nerve tension. As reflexology encourages the body to relax, other functions are affected. Every part of the body receives its nerve supply from the spine. Abnormal tension causes tightening of the muscles of the spine; thus nerves are affected, resulting in pain. When tension is relaxed, the muscles cease to contract. Blood vessels too are relaxed, reducing vascular constriction and allowing circulation to flow freely, thereby conducting the necessary oxygen and nutrients to all the body tissues and organs. This in turn helps cleanse the body of toxins and impurities.

Stress is difficult to avoid. It is an integral part of modern life. The days when the stress syndrome was associated only with high-powered business executives are long gone. Today young children, women, men and the elderly are all subject to varying degrees of stress. Survival in the twentieth century is stressful. The rapid pace and modern technology contribute to major malfunctions in body and psyche. The barrage of 'stressors' is unrelenting – traffic, television, noise, job pressure, family problems, wars, famines, disease, environmental problems, electronic smog, financial problems, global problems, pollution – the list is endless.

Few people escape the consequences of stress. The increasing number of people with heart disease and high blood pressure is evidence of the more obvious stress-related diseases. Other symptoms, though more nebulous, can also be deadly. Long-term symptoms of constant exposure to stress are fatigue, anxiety and depression. The nervous system becomes drained and depleted, and the immune system eroded, making one more susceptible to immuno-deficiency diseases.

Not all stress is negative. It can be immensely stimulating. The human body is equipped to cope with short-term invigorating stress. But long-term constant exposure to stress is devastating.

Stress affects different people in different ways and to varying degrees. One person may exhibit cardiovascular problems, another gastro-intestinal upset, anorexia, palpitations, sweating or headaches – to mention but a few of the myriad body reactions. The cardiovascular and digestive systems are targets for the ill-effects of stress – high blood pressure, ulcers and indigestion being obvious results. Stress can also be linked to infectious diseases. When the body is busy dealing with the effects of residual stress, it cannot organize an effective defence against invading organisms.[6]

Reflexology helps to alleviate the effects of stress by inducing deep relaxation, thereby allowing the nervous system to function normally and free the body to seek its own homeostasis. Reflexology is a powerful antidote to stress. A relaxed body can heal itself and reflexology is a guaranteed method of relaxing the body and balancing the biological systems. For hypertension and anxiety, choose reflexology rather than tranquillizers – it is a safe way to induce relaxation and has no unpleasant side-effects.

REFLEXOLOGY AND THE NERVOUS SYSTEM

The nervous system is the body's 'electrical' system, and the most complex system of the body. Without a nerve supply the organs of the body could not function. Every part of the body is operated by messages carried back and forth along neural pathways. The nervous system is divided into three parts; the central nervous system, the peripheral nervous system, and the autonomic nervous system. It is believed that nerve impulses initiated through pressure on the reflexes of the feet *may* be connected to the autonomic nervous system.

The autonomic nervous system controls the involuntary action of internal organs, muscles and glands. There are two parts to the system – the sympathetic and parasympathetic. These parts have opposing effects on the body. They both send out weak impulses to the organs and glands to maintain normal activity. However, in stressful situations, the sympathetic impulses become stronger and the organs and glands react to the situation. The parasympathetic system takes over when the stress has passed and returns the body functions to normal.

Many reflexologists believe that stimulating the reflex areas of the feet has an effect on the internal organs via a simple reflex action. A reflex is an unconscious or involuntary response to a stimulus. Some reflex actions are quite common and simple, such as the pupil of the eye reacting to light, or the jerk of the leg when the knee is tapped. For a reflex action to occur there must first be a stimulus. In the case of reflexology, the stimulus is provided when pressure is applied to the reflex areas of the feet. This activates an electro-chemical nerve impulse which is conducted to the central nervous system via a sensory (afferent) neurone. This message is received by the ganglion and then transmitted via a motor (efferent) neurone which then causes a response.

The autonomic nervous system does not work apart from the rest of the nervous system. A loud noise perceived by the sensory system can speed up the beating of the heart, thereby influencing the entire circulatory system. A chronic state of worry or excitement involving a voluntary part of the nervous system will often result in pathological conditions involving the autonomic part of the nervous system.[7]

The neural pathways are both living tissue and electrical channels and can be impinged upon or polluted by many factors. When neural pathways are impaired nerve function is impeded – messages are delivered slowly and unreliably, and body processes operate at less than optimum levels. Reflexology, by stimulating the thousands of nerve endings in the feet, encourages the opening and clearing of neural pathways.

REFLEXOLOGY AND CIRCULATION

One of Eunice Ingham's favourite sayings was: 'Circulation is life. Stagnation is death.' Every practitioner acknowledges the importance of good circulation. If the smallest fraction of circulation is cut off from one or more parts of the body, the effects soon become evident in a variety of aches and pains. All the tissues of the body depend on an adequate blood supply to function properly and the application of reflexology benefits the body circulation.

Blood carries oxygen and nutrients to the cells and removes waste products and toxins. During this process, blood vessels contract and relax so their resilience is most important for proper functioning. Stress and tension tighten up the cardiovascular system and restrict blood flow. Circulation becomes sluggish, causing high or low blood pressure.

The increased state of relaxation facilitated by reflexology allows the body systems – including the excretory systems – to function efficiently, eliminating toxins and impurities properly. By reducing stress and tension, reflexology allows the cardiovascular vessels to conduct the flow of blood naturally and easily.

Circulatory factors *are* influenced by the pressure applied in reflexology. The effects of reflexology on blood pressure have been proven in a blood pressure study at the California Police Olympics, where reflexologists participated in 'demonstration' booths during the 1987 games. A small informal blood pressure study was conducted by the Sacramento Valley Reflexology Association. It was found that reflexology normalized (either brought it up or down, as needed) the systolic pressure in 75 per cent and the diastolic pressure in 61 per cent of those cases studied.[8]

REFLEXOLOGY AND THE ENDOCRINE SYSTEM

If the nerves are considered the 'electrical' system of the body, then the endocrine glands are the 'chemical' system. The endocrine system is an intricate network of glands which secrete hormones on which every bodily activity is dependent directly into the blood. Hormones are extremely powerful chemical substances. If any one of the seven principal glands is out of order, hormone secretion will be disrupted and the whole body thrown off balance.

An important gland, the pancreas, provides an excellent example of the intricacy of body balancing. One of its main functions is to maintain the balance of glucose or blood sugar. This is achieved with the hormone insulin, which activates the body cells to take up the glucose from the blood. The body cells or tissues break this down into carbon dioxide and water to produce energy and it is stored by the liver as glycogen. Without insulin, the glucose is not consumed or is stored improperly. It accumulates in the blood causing the dangerous condition diabetes. If excess insulin is produced, the opposite effect occurs. When insulin removes glucose from the blood by increased combustion, the storage of glucose in the form of glycogen is increased at the expense of the blood.

Low blood sugar (hypoglycaemia) is the result. The balance has been disrupted.[9]

Every tissue and organ in the body is controlled by the complex interaction among chemicals circulating in the blood stream and the hormones secreted by the glands. The hormones secreted by the *anterior* part of the pituitary gland, often referred to as the master gland of the body, are under the influence of the hypothalamus. Recent research has shown that nerves connect the thymus and spleen directly to the hypothalamus which affects the immune system. In essence, the brain controls the immune system just as it does with pain control and the production of endorphins (strong pain-killing proteins occurring naturally in the brain).[10]

Thoughts and emotions are affected by the glands, and personality is determined by gland function. If gland function is harmonious, one will have a positive happy outlook; disharmonious functioning will cause a depressive outlook. Reflexology, by stimulating the electrical energy, has a subsidiary effect on the chemical energy.

REFLEXOLOGY AND PAIN CONTROL

A number of chemical changes take place in the body during reflexology treatment. One such change deals with the sedation of pain. The body produces its own pain-killers, known as endorphins, which are five to ten times more powerful than morphine. Endorphins are produced by the pituitary gland and can inhibit the transmission of pain signals through the spinal cord.

Studies have revealed that pain signals travel along the nerve pathways to the dorsal horn of the spinal cord, beginning a complicated reflex action. From the spinal cord the impulse is relayed to the thalamus, where the sensations of heat, cold, pain and touch are recognized. The thalamus forwards the impulse along to the cerebral cortex where the intensity and location of the pain is recognized. The brain then sends signals back through the spinal cord to release endorphins. However, according to the 'gate control theory', the nervous system can only respond to a limited amount of sensory information at one time. When the system becomes overloaded it short-circuits, or closes a gate, reducing the amount of sensory information available for processing. The application of reflexology encourages the brain to produce more endorphins while the pressure also acts to confuse the body with too many sensations to respond to, forcing the body to close the 'pain gates'.[11] This interrupts the pain cycle, eases pain and helps the body to relax.[12]

REFLEXOLOGY AND TERMINAL DISEASES

In cases of terminal illness such as cancer, multiple sclerosis and AIDS, reflexology may not be capable of removing the cause of the disease but it does make the patient more comfortable and the pain more bearable. It can significantly improve the patient's general condition, activate excretory organs, stimulate the respiratory system and help the patient achieve better control of bladder and bowels. Reflexology can, thereby, improve the quality of life. With AIDS, reflexology can work on the immune system, helping to prolong life.

REFLEXOLOGY AND CRYSTAL DEPOSITS

Grainy crystal deposits, which cause pain during treatment, may be felt in the nerve endings of the feet. These are believed to be calcium deposits which have settled beneath the skin surface at the nerve endings. Excess acidity in the bloodstream increases calcium deposits in the nerve endings of any organ in the body. These deposits develop into acid crystals which can impede normal blood circulation. The feet are a prime target of these congestions because of the abundance of nerve endings present here, and the fact that feet are usually restricted in shoes preventing the natural movement of the foot. Thus the normal nerve and blood supply to the feet is slowed down. The feet are also at the end point of circulation and blood has to be circulated back up against the force of gravity. Congestion will impede this function, and toxins will tend to stagnate in the feet. These crystals can be broken down by reflexology massage and the residue removed by the blood circulation.

WHO CAN BENEFIT FROM REFLEXOLOGY?

Reflexology does not discriminate. There are no boundaries or limitations. People of any age or sex – the elderly, women, men, teenagers, children and babies – can derive positive benefits from reflexology. Reflexology can do no harm although please remember that caution should be taken with thrombosis (it could move the blood clot), and with diabetes, especially if insulin is being given (if the treatment activates the pancreas the insulin level has to be reduced). Other restrictions are those determined by the receiver's pain threshold and their reactions to massage. Elderly people with no specific complaint will benefit from a couple of courses of treatment a year to keep bodily functions toned. Results are also good with children and babies because they are more relaxed and supple and because their bodies are highly receptive to therapeutic stimuli.

Reflexology has proved itself to be effective, but because no two people are the same, what may be of great benefit for one person may not have the same results for another. Because reflexology treatment reaches the receiver on several levels – physical, mental and spiritual – it can only be of benefit.

SPIRITUAL SYMBOLISM

Our feet also play a significant role in our spiritual well-being. Our feet connect us to the ground and they are therefore a connection between our earthly and spiritual life. They ground us literally and figuratively. They are our base and foundation and our contact with the earth and the energies that flow through it.

The importance of feet was recognized in Biblical times (John 13: 2–10): 'And the supper being ended, the devil having now put him into the heart of Judas Iscariot, Simon's son, to betray him; Jesus, knowing that the father had given all things into his hands, and that he was come from God and went to God; He riseth from supper and laid aside his garments; and took a towel and girded himself. After that he poureth water into a basin, and began to wash his disciples' feet, and to wipe them with the towel wherewith he was girded. Then cometh he to Simon Peter; and Peter saith unto him; Lord dost thou wash my feet? Jesus answered him, if I wash thee not thou hast no part with me. Simon Peter saith unto him, Lord, not my feet only, but also my hands and head. Jesus saith to him, He that is washed needeth not save to wash his feet but is clean every whit.'

In his writings, Omraam Mikhäel Aïvanhov draws interesting symbolic connections between the feet and the solar plexus in relation to astrology, Christian teachings and the miracle of the five loaves and fishes. 'Every religion comes under the influence of two constellations diametrically opposite each other on the zodiacal circle. The Christian religion comes under the influence of Pisces (the fishes) and its polar opposite Virgo (the Virgin) and we find references to these two symbols in the Gospels.'[13]

'Each part of our body is related to one of the constellations: Aries – head; Taurus – neck; Gemini – arms and lungs; Cancer – stomach; Leo – heart; Virgo – intestines and solar plexus; Libra – kidneys; Scorpio – genital organs; Sagittarius – thighs; Capricorn – knees; Aquarius – calves; Pisces – feet. Astrology tells us that it is the solar plexus that is in relation to Virgo and the feet to Pisces. Since Virgo and Pisces are connected and represent the axis of Christ, there must also be a connection between the feet and the solar plexus.

'The solar plexus is a part of the sympathetic nerve system which is a network of nerve fibres, ganglia and plexuses. It is located just behind the stomach and consists of five ordinary ganglia and two so-called 'half-moon' ganglia shaped like fishes. These are the five loaves and the two fishes,

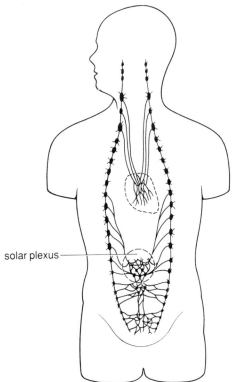

solar plexus

Fig.3 The solar plexus and the half-moon ganglia

the male and the female united in the solar plexus.

'As long as a child is in its mother's womb it is bound to her by the umbilical cord through which it receives the nourishment it needs. The mother represents Nature. When a child is separated from the mother at birth the umbilical cord is cut, but there is another invisible cord which connects every child to Mother Nature who continues to nourish it. And this cord must not be cut until man is fully equipped to live his separate life, for man is a child of Nature and if the cord is cut prematurely he will no longer receive the nourishment he needs and will die. Astrology tells us that this invisible cord links man to Nature, his mother, through the solar plexus.

'The two half-moon ganglia enable man to move through space at will and the five ordinary ganglia are the five loaves with which the multitude of his cells are nourished. Each ganglion is related to one of the five virtues symbolised by the pentagram; kindness, justice, love, wisdom and truth. Mercury, the ruler of Virgo, is represented in the Gospel story by the young boy who brought the loaves and fishes which Jesus multiplied and distributed to the multitude. And the five thousand are all the cells that make up the physical body and which receive their daily nourishment from the solar plexus . . .

'The loaves and fishes which were multiplied by Jesus were not ordinary material loaves and fishes . . . The account of the miracle by which Jesus multiplied the loaves and fishes to feed five thousand is symbolic and should not be understood literally. In each of us the solar plexus feeds thousands upon thousands of cells with its five loaves and two fishes . . . Every human being has a solar plexus, but most of them are so bogged down in material things and their lives are so chaotic that the solar plexus cannot do its own subtle work. Every human being possesses five loaves and two fishes, but the great majority are not properly nourished; they nourish themselves on the physical plane without realising that they also need spiritual food.'[14]

Aïvanhov goes on to take this theory even further. 'The Christian era was under the influence of Pisces and its opposite sign Virgo. Jesus was born of the Virgin, and he himself represents Pisces, the fish. In washing of the feet we shall once again find this Virgo-Pisces polarity, but from another point of view.

'According to the astrological tradition, there is a correspondence between man's feet and the constellation of Pisces and between the solar plexus and Virgo. If Jesus washed his disciples' feet it was in order to show them the extremely important link between the feet and the solar plexus.

'Of course it is true that with the gesture it was as though Jesus was telling his disciples, "This is an example I am giving you. Later on you too will have to show the same humility and unselfishness towards others." And he then washed Judas' feet although he knew perfectly well that Judas had already betrayed him. Symbolically you could say that someone who refuses to take revenge on those who have done him a wrong, washes their feet. But Jesus' gesture was, above all, intended to awaken in his disciples the constructive energies of the solar plexus. The seven main chakras repeat themselves in reverse order from the coccyx down to the feet. With this esoteric theory the Crown chakra is represented on the soles of the feet. The Christ washed the disciples' feet in order to awaken the Crown Chakra above the head, to awaken the spiritual energies.

'Probably in the ordinary circumstances of daily life, some of you have already noticed a connection between your feet and your solar plexus. When your feet are cold you can feel a tightening of the solar plexus, and if you eat while you're feeling like that, your digestion will be more difficult than usual. But you will find that if you soak your feet in hot water it will give you a delightful sensation of relaxation at the level of your solar plexus and you will feel on top of your form. That is why, if you are feeling anxious or tense, I advise you to consciously and deliberately prepare a basin of hot water, to soak your feet in it and wash them with attention: in this way you will be influencing and strengthening your solar plexus and your state of consciousness will immediately be transformed . . .

'We must never forget that it is by means of our feet that we maintain the contact with the earth and its telluric currents: they serve as antennae. But the electro-magnetic currents arising from the earth or flowing down into it can only circulate freely if the feet are not charged with layers of fluidic impurities; that is why it is good to wash one's feet every evening.

'To begin with Peter refused to let Jesus wash his feet and later he asked him to wash not only his feet but his head and hands as well, and Jesus told him: "He that is washed needeth not save to wash his feet, but is clean every whit." The feet being the part of the body which is most closely in contact with the earth, they represent the physical plane which we have to transcend in order to gain access to higher planes, and this is why if we consciously fix our attention on and under our feet while we are washing them, we can work towards this liberation from the physical plane . . .

'The feet therefore symbolise the physical sphere and of course it is in the physical sphere that we are always victimised since the feet symbolise the most material, to wash one's feet represents the final touch in the work of purification . . .

'So, as you can see, Jesus' gesture in washing his disciples' feet has a much deeper significance than is usually realised . . . Begin to work on your feet and your solar plexus on a spiritual level and you will soon feel very beneficial results.'[15]

Section two

THE HOLISTIC APPROACH

Disease (is) not an entity but a fluctuating condition of the patient's body, a battle between the substance of disease and the natural self-healing tendency of the body.

HIPPOCRATES

HOLISM is a recently rediscovered concept in healing. According to the holistic approach to medicine, health is defined as a positive, glowing state of mental and physical well-being, not merely the absence of disease. Prior to the advent of modern medicine the manifestation of disease was recognized as being the result of disharmony in the physical, emotional and spiritual spheres, and health perceived as a balance between these three. Thus no symptom or disorder could be treated in isolation. Holistic healing methods, therefore, always treat the person as a whole. They do not work specifically on an impaired organ or malfunctioning system, but on the whole person with the aim of mobilizing the body's own healing powers to restore the organism to a state of equilibrium.

People in the West take their health for granted and abuse it in many different ways. Eventually the system breaks down, sickness and disease arise, and they wonder why. For thousands of years it was accepted that illness resulted from a disturbance in man's internal environment. Then came the orthodox scientific approach dominated by the germ theory. This theory evolved from the findings of French chemist and biologist Louis Pasteur, the founder of bacteriology. It has been the focus of medicine ever since. Once it was known that micro-organisms could invade the body and flourish into specific diseases, the search was on to seek out, identify and combat them.[1] Man came to be perceived as a sum of working parts and the approach to disease dominated by symptomatic diagnosis and palliative treatment.

The germ theory has been quite convenient, as most of us prefer to believe that illness is the result of external forces. This approach is now seen to be far too simplistic. The failure of the germ theory to combat the vast and intricate realm of disease has resulted in increased interest in, and demand for, natural therapies; therapies which recognize that the problem of health and disease does not lie in identifying symptoms but in the greater understanding of people and their needs as individuals.

Micro-organisms may be involved in many ailments but their presence does not automatically guarantee disease. We are constantly surrounded by numerous disease-bearing organisms in the environment, but only a fraction of the people exposed to these succumb to any form of infection. For example, if three people breathe the same germs at the same time, one may develop pneumonia, another a cold, and the third may never be aware that the germs were there.

Disease is generated by a combination of circumstances both inside and outside the body. The main object of holistic healing is to help correct the life condition that predisposes a person to disease. A vast number of factors can initiate disease – particularly in our modern, highly industrialized, polluted environment. Yet one of the most important factors in the development of disease is state of mind.

The mind is immensely powerful and the relationship between mind and body should never be underestimated. Because all life is based on energy, health is considered to be the harmonious interplay of energies within the body. Negative thoughts and emotions restrict the free flow of these energies, causing congestions which ultimately manifest as disease if not corrected. It is now widely accepted that a positive attitude is a major step towards creating a healthy body. This is most eloquently expressed by Dr Randolph Stone who said: 'As you think, so you are.' He wrote in *Health Building*: 'We become what we contemplate. Negative thoughts and fears make grooves in the mind as negative energy waves of despondency and hopelessness. We cannot think negative thoughts and reap positive results, and therefore we must assert the positive and maintain a positive pattern of thinking and acting as our ideals.'[2]

All thoughts and emotions reverberate throughout every cell in the body and manifest physiologically. For example, the angry and disturbed person develops an acid system, a preponderance of the positively charged H^+ ion.[3] Emotions also alter endocrine balance, impair blood supply and blood pressure, impede digestion, change body temperature and produce a sustained state of emotional stress, causing physiological changes that lead to disease.[4]

Illness is a natural expression of what is happening inside the body. It is pointless to treat this with superficial drugs designed to suppress the problem, as the seat of the disease may be in a different part of the body from the one in which it manifests.

The human body is composed of about 1000 billion cells all working towards a common end – the maintenance of a healthy individual.[5] These body cells are constantly changing. The materials of our bodies and brains are renewed regularly. All the protein in the body is replaced every six months and in some organs, such as the liver, the protein is renewed more frequently.[6]

We acquire a new stomach lining every five days (the innermost layer of stomach cells is exchanged in a matter of minutes as food is digested). Skin is new every five weeks. The skeleton is entirely new every three months.

Every year 98 per cent of the total number of atoms in the body are replaced.[7] And at the end of each seven-year period, every cell in the body has been replaced. This raises an interesting question. How do the cells 'know' what form to take? This is where Dr Harold Saxton Burr's life-field comes into play. Says Burr: 'When we meet a friend we have not seen for six months there is not one molecule in his face which was there when we last saw him. But thanks to his controlling L-field, the new molecules have fallen into the old, familiar pattern and we can recognise his face. Until modern instruments revealed the existence of the controlling L-field, biologists were at a loss to explain how our bodies "keep in shape" through ceaseless metabolism and changes of material. Now the mystery has been solved. The electro-dynamic field of the body serves as a matrix or mould, which preserves the "shape" or arrangement of any mat-erial poured into it, however often the material may be changed.'[8]

If the cells in the body are turning over at such a rapid rate, it should be possible to replace tired, burnt out, unhealthy cells with new, vibrant, healthy cells, thereby creating a 'new' body imbued with vitality. As old cells die and disappear, instead of replacing them with cells programmed with the same negative thoughts and fed on inadequate nutrition, one should learn to re-programme them with positive, nutritious information to create a 'new' being. This is not impossible. It just requires dedic-ated effort and the genuine desire for health.

It does, however, seem that in the modern world we face almost insurmountable odds. Rapid industrialization, modern technology and the rapid pace of modern society combined with disintegration of moral values has resulted in man moving away from working in accord-ance with the natural laws of the universe. This is causing widespread disease in the body and psyche of the delicate human organism. Modern medicine may have managed to control many infectious diseases once considered life-threatening, but we are now faced with a gamut of 'new' diseases that are baffling modern medi-cine. Diseases like cancer, AIDS, myalgic en-cephalomyelitis (ME) and birth defects are on the increase throughout the Western indus-trialized world. While AIDS was called the 'disease of the 80s', ME is now seen as the disease of the 90s. And there are no cures in sight. Both afflictions are related to the immune system, and the immune system suffers most from constant exposure to stress. Could the stress of modern living be killing us?

Major psychological diseases are also on the increase – for example, depression, and the com-pulsive use of legal and illegal drugs, ranging from caffeine, nicotine, alchohol and prescrip-tion drugs to marijuana, cocaine, heroin and 'crack'. These are symptoms of an unhealthy society. And as we rush towards the twenty-first century with our indiscriminate 'advances' in technology, we are creating an environment that is becoming increasingly hostile to human life. If we continue to pollute our environment, the world will soon be irreversibly damaged, and so too the physical, mental and spiritual health of all the planet's inhabitants.

Every person has the potential for perfect health. It may require effort and dedication, but the rewards are tremendous. To quote Dr Stone: 'Health is not merely of the body. It is the natural expression of the body, mind and soul when they are in rhythm with the One Life. True Health is the harmony of life within us, consisting of peace of mind, happiness and well-being. It is not merely a question of physical fitness, but it is rather the result of the soul finding free expression through the mind and body of that individual. Such a person radiates peace and happiness and everyone in his presence automatically feels happy and contented.'[9]

CHAPTER ONE

Energies

Someone once asked the question:
'What is this electricity which constitutes a field?'
A distinguished physicist gave the best answer that the author knows: 'Electricity
is the way Nature behaves.'
This electricity then, which can be measured and shown to have order and pattern,
is not some strange and separate phenomenon, but an essential characteristic of the
Universe.

DR HAROLD SAXTON BURR

As energy is an important facet in this approach to reflexology it is imperative that one has some understanding of the effects of external energies – both natural and manmade – on the human body and mind. All living creatures possess the same common denominator – electromagnetic energy. Everything in the universe is linked by energy fields, creating an intricate web of inter-dependence.

Our planet is a vibrant, pulsating mass of energy which lives and breathes in accordance with the natural laws of the universe. We as living organisms inhabiting this sphere are in turn electromagnetically intertwined with the energies of the earth. Our biological cycles are regulated by the earth's electromagnetic field; thus we are affected by changes in this field. The earth's field varies in response to the moon and the sun, so these too have an effect on us. To understand a little more of how these cosmic occurrences affect life, we'll look briefly at the earth, sun and moon.

EARTH

The earth's electromagnetic field is the result of interaction between the planet's molten nickel-iron core and the charged gas of the ionosphere.[1] This field is influenced by changes in lunar and solar events and it has a profound effect on life on the planet.

How are we as humans related to this? Over the years researchers have come up with some very interesting information. First is that the earth's magnetic field fluctuates between eight and sixteen times each second – the same as the prominent rhythm of our brain.[2] Also, the frequency of the micropulsations of the field is the prime timer of our biological cycles. Studies of the pineal gland have proved this. The pineal gland, situated in the centre of the cranium, produces melatonin and seratonin, two neuro-hormones that (among many other functions) directly control all the biocycles. Small magnetic fields influence the pineal gland – either increasing or decreasing production of melatonin and seratonin.[3]

The reason for this could be magnetic attraction. Magnetic deposits have been discovered close to the pineal and pituitary glands in the sinuses of the ethmoid bone, the spongy bone in the centre of the head behind the nose and between the eyes. It is possible that this transmits the biocycle timing cues from the earth field's micropulsations to the pineal gland.[4]

To further illustrate the point, it has been proved that the L-fields described by Harold Saxton Burr register changes in response to sunlight, darkness, cycles of the moon, magnetic storms and sun-spots. This was discovered by testing the fields on trees – an excellent 'subject' as they live to a great age and do not move about, so can be attached to equipment for extended periods. The fact that extraterrestrial forces have such a profound impact on the L-field of trees indicates that they would probably have a more pronounced impact on the complex L-field of humans.[5]

SUN

Energy for all life on earth depends on the sun. But this solar energy is not always positive. Man's body functions are subject to some fairly extreme responses to sun-induced changes in the earth's magnetic field. One of the most disruptive effects of the sun is sun-spot activity. This occurs in eleven-year cycles and can be equated with nuclear explosions on the face of the sun, which emit a barrage of electro-magnetic vibrations that bombard the earth. These solar disturbances can be related to major

events on earth, and have been known to coincide with social problems, wars and epidemics. Sun-spot activity was occurring at the time of the Black Death in England, great plagues, diphtheria and cholera outbreaks in Europe, the Russian typhus and smallpox epidemics.[6] And the last six peaks of the eleven-year sun-spot cycle have coincided with major flu epidemics.

Dr Robert Becker discovered correlations between disturbances in the earth's field caused by magnetic storms on the sun emitting 'cosmic rays' and the rate of psychiatric admissions. He found that significantly more people were signed in to psychiatric services just after magnetic disturbances than when the field was stable. He also found a similar influence on schizophrenic patients who exhibited behaviour changes one or two days after cosmic ray decreases, due to low energy cosmic ray flares from the sun which produce strong disruptions in the earth's field one or two days after the magnetic storms.[7]

MOON

The moon, too, has a profound influence on us. The earth attracts the moon strongly enough to hold it in its orbit – and all bodies of water on the earth, both large and small, are affected by the moon. As the human body is made up of approximately 75 per cent water, it is obvious that we too would be directly affected by the moon.

The moon affects conception and optimizes fertility levels. The average length of the menstrual cycle is almost identical to the time between two full moons. In some places the moon is referred to as 'the great midwife'. Research conducted in New York hospitals between 1948 and 1957 showed a trend for more births to take place during the waning moon than the waxing moon with a maximum just after the full moon and a clear minimum at new moon.[8]

It has also been noted that bleeding is greater at the time when the moon is increasing. In an article entitled 'The Moon and You' which appeared in *This Week* magazine during 1968, the author tells of the experience of Dr Edson Andrews of Florida. After his nurse called attention to the fact that bleeding increased at full moon, he checked the records and discovered that during this time more patients had to be returned to the operating room following surgery. A later study of a thousand cases revealed to Dr Andrews that 82 per cent of the bleeding crises occurred between 'third and first' phases of the moon. Nearly all attacks of bleeding ulcers came when the moon was full.[9] It was also reported that haemorrhages occur chiefly at full moon, which has subsequently been supported by scientific proof.

The connection between the moon and madness has long been acknowledged – as is implied by the term 'lunacy'. The American Institute of Climatology has published a report on the effect of a full moon on human behaviour in which it records that crimes with strong psychotic motivation, such as arson, kleptomania, destructive driving and homicidal alchoholism all show marked peaks when the moon is full.[10]

The earth's electromagnetic activity obviously has profound effects on life. So what of the effects of the artificial, man-made energies? We have radically distorted our electromagnetic environment in the few decades since World War II. We are now completely surrounded by a sea of strange energies – the consequences of which we are only now beginning to discover.

Modern life revolves around electronic gizmos and gadgets. In the Western world, no home or office could function without a generous supply of 'equipment': radios, televisions, com- ͏ters, digital watches, microwave ovens,

stereos, electronic locking systems, fridges, ovens, telephones, radar, electric trains, CB radios, electric blankets, and anti-theft devices. Before the advent of electricity, radio, telephones and other electronic 'advances', the earth was quiet, and all organisms were regulated by the natural influences of the earth and nature. Today the world is a network of abnormal fields – the radio waves around us alone are now 100 to 200 million times the natural level reaching us from the sun.[11] These manmade fields are producing abnormalities in human and animal responses.

Electromagnetic radiation (EMR) encompasses an enormous range of frequencies – gamma rays, X-rays, ultraviolet wavelengths, infra-red waves, microwaves (those we've harnessed for communication) and radio waves which are broken down from extremely high to extremely low frequencies. It is the extremely low frequencies (ELF) which seem most damaging to human health.[12]

Let us look at the effects of fields most people are exposed to in their normal home and office environments.

Research was conducted using ELF fields to simulate normal background levels of a typical office. When rats were exposed to this field, levels of the neurotransmitter acetylcholine in the brainstem increased. This activated a subliminal distress signal, without the animal being aware of it.[13]

Monkeys exposed to ELF electric fields roughly equivalent to the field from a colour TV set sixty feet away exhibited changes in response times.[14] All video display units (VDUs) including video games, televisions and computer monitors emit varying amounts of radiation over a broad spectrum. The transformers release very low frequency and extremely low frequency waves, while microwaves, X-rays and ultraviolet waves emanate from the screen. Many VDU operators suffer headaches, nausea, neck and back pain, and vision impairment. VDUs have also been linked to miscarriages, stillbirths, embryonic deformities and birth defects among pregnant women working in computerized offices. Embryo deformities could be the result of chromosomal damage caused by electromagnetic radiation.[15]

Energy depletion and constant fatigue are recognized symptoms of excess exposure to VDUs. Look at the 'couch potato' syndrome. How many people spend the majority of their time slumped in front of the TV screen? And the increase in computer-crazy kids? Could this be electromagnetic addiction? As the body becomes accustomed to having its polarities reversed or energies disharmonized, it craves the continuance of the process. It becomes a vicious circle and a hard habit to break.[16]

Even something as simple as the common old telephone disrupts our energy fields. The brain has a weak magnetic field. Davis and Rawls in the '60s and '70s pointed out that the powerful cobalt samarian magnets used in telephones can detrimentally affect the functioning of the brain whenever the earpiece is held close to the head. Electric hairdryers, shavers and the like also produce electromagnetic fields and radiation which are bound to interact with brainwave patterns and brain functions.[17]

Rats exposed to low level microwaves similar to mealtime exposure from microwave ovens exhibited metabolic changes: changes of liver functions; vitamin B2 and B6 depletion from blood, brain, liver, kidneys and heart; and major shifts in trace metal metabolism.[18]

Subliminal activation of the stress response is one of the most significant effects electromagnetic frequencies and non-ionizing radiation have on life, but it is not the only one. These unfamiliar energies produce changes in nearly every bodily function so far studied.

SUBLIMINAL STRESS

In Russian research on rats, administration of steady magnetic fields caused cell death in the brain, and generalized stress reaction marked by large amounts of cortisone in the blood-stream. This is a 'slow' stress response evident in prolonged stress, not the 'fight-or-flight' response generated by adrenaline. Cortisone levels in monkeys exposed to a magnetic field for four hours a day showed stress response for six days when it subsided. This suggested adaption to the field – but this tolerance of continued stress is illusory.

Dr Hans Selye, in his pioneering life work on stress, explains that, initially, stress activates the hormonal and/or immune systems to a higher than normal level, enabling the animal to escape danger or combat disease. If the stress continues, hormone levels and immune reactivity gradually decline to normal. However, if the stressful condition persists, hormone and immune levels decline further, well below normal. In medical terms stress *decompensation* has set in and the animal is now more susceptible to other stressors, including malignant growth and infectious diseases.[19]

Electropollution can trigger radical and dangerous changes. These dangers are very real. Most people are subject to extremely high daily exposure, particularly in cities which are subject to a whole spectrum of frequencies from ELF to microwave. The greatest danger lies in uncontrolled exposure to large amounts of electromagnetic radiation at many overlapping frequencies.[20] All cities, by their very nature as electrical centres, are jungles of interpenetrating fields and radiation that completely drown out the earth's background throb.[21] All life pulsates in time to the earth but the natural rhythms have now been overwhelmed by artificial fields, which can have drastic repercussions in all organisms. Even the changing weather patterns we are witnessing globally could be partially attributed to electropollution. We are treading on dangerous ground.

Says Dr Becker: 'The ultimate weapon is manipulation of the electromagnetic environment, because it is imperceptibly subtle and strikes at the very core of life itself. We're dealing here with the most important scientific discovery ever – the nature of life. Even if we survive the chemical and atomic threats of our existence, there's a strong possibility that increasing electropollution could set in motion irreversible changes leading to our extinction before we're even aware of them.'[22]

When confronted with this kind of evidence, it may seem we're trying to fight a losing battle. How can we ever achieve health when we're being bombarded by an enemy we cannot perceive? However, the correct effort to strengthen our own energy fields and state of health will increase our ability to cope with the additional stresses of electropollution.

CHAPTER TWO

Stress

The mass of men lead lives of quiet desperation.
HENRY DAVID THOREAU

Stress is probably one of the most commonly used words in today's society but stress is not new to the human condition. It has always been present, but is now more prevalent as the pressure and demands of the twentieth century take their toll. The word 'stress' is derived from the Latin word *stringere* which means 'to draw tight'. The modern word 'uptight' accurately describes the response to stress.

The stress reaction is a primitive response to a threatening or dangerous situation, and has been of essential importance in ensuring the continued survival of the human species. Man is the product of thousands of years of evolution. His survival has depended on quick physical responses to dangers and the stress reaction is commonly referred to as the 'fight-or-flight' reaction.

In primitive times, this burst of energy was utilized in physical activity such as a life-or-death struggle or a quick dash to safety. Today these responses are largely unacceptable. To attack the boss or a shop assistant for causing you stress would invariably result in legal repercussions, while fleeing from a tense meeting would be perceived as a mental aberration.

Until recently it was believed that all stress was a result of external forces exerting pressure on an individual. This does not explain why, when confronted by similar situations, one person will react calmly while another may be completely devastated. More recent theories emphasize that the stress response depends on the interaction between a person and his or her environment. The intensity of the stress experience is determined by how a person feels he or she can cope with an identified threat.

The hormonal and chemical defence mechanisms that evolved over the centuries as a means of protection have been retained, but today they have little outlet. The inability to express any physical response to a stressful situation means that our natural instincts are suppressed, which can cause dire harm.

What exactly are the physiological effects of stress? When confronted by a situation we perceive as threatening, our thoughts regarding ourselves and the situation trigger two branches of the central nervous system – the sympathetic and parasympathetic systems.

The sympathetic nervous system initiates involuntary responses designed to activate all the major systems of the body. The first response is a flood of hormone secretions. The hypothalamus, when recognizing a danger, triggers the pituitary gland. This gland releases hormones which cause the adrenal glands to intensify the output of adrenaline and noradrenaline into the bloodstream. These two hormones mimic the actions of nervous stimulation in a number of organs in the body. Although any number of factors can trigger the adrenocortical stress reaction, the response itself is always the same. It involves the release from the adrenal glands of specific hormones, mainly the corticosteroids, which in turn mobilize the body against invading germs or foreign proteins and enhance one's level of arousal. The stress response always activates the immune system.

The stress chemicals induce physiological changes designed to improve performance. Blood supply to the brain is increased, initially improving judgement and decision making. The heart speeds up and fuel is released into the bloodstream from glucose, fats or stored blood sugar to provide additional energy. More blood is sent to the muscles to allow for instant action. Breathing rate and function improve as air passages relax. A sense of stimulation is produced and blood pressure rises. Because digestion and excretion are not considered high priorities in a 'dangerous' situation, adrenaline causes vascular constriction which reduces the flow of blood to the stomach and intestine. Blood vessels dilate in some areas and constrict in others; for example, blood is drained from the skin to make it available for use in other areas like the muscles.

When the body prepares for 'fight-or-flight', it is ready for a short burst of heightened activity. In modern society numerous factors can trigger this response, but few can be dealt with by a short burst of activity. Often stress situations are continuous so stress responses are semi-permanently on red-alert, but physical release is usually unacceptable, so this is all suppressed – a situation which cannot be maintained for too long. The stress build-up eventually explodes internally, knocks the body systems out of balance and causes extreme physical and mental exhaustion.

The role of the parasympathetic nervous system is to relax the body after a stressful encounter. However, if a person is subject to continuous stress, it becomes more difficult to activate the parasympathetic reaction. If the stress situation continues unabated, the body weakens and becomes more susceptible to a variety of diseases.

Long-term adrenal stimulation with no discharge of energy will deplete essential minerals and vitamins from the system, for example Vitamins B and C, which are vital for the functioning of the immune system.[1] This will result in lowered resistance and increased susceptibility to diseases directly related to the immune system like AIDS and ME. Long-term adrenal accumulation can also affect blood pressure and cause a build-up of fatty substances on blood vessel walls, as well as damaging the functioning of the digestive system.

When an organism must face a continual or repeated stress, the response system enters the chronic phase, during which resistance declines below normal and eventually becomes exhausted. Several diseases result directly from this stage, but the most important effect is a decrease in the body's ability to fight infection and cancer.[2]

Everyone is confronted daily with potentially stressful situations. One's vulnerability to stress can be influenced by life events which cause undue emotional strain. Emotional distress is one resistance-lowering factor. Another important factor, according to some health professionals, is the impact of major life changes. Virtually all illness is preceded by a constellation of significant events in our lives. Future health or disease can be forecast by evaluating these events. The greater the number of life changes, the more serious the oncoming illness.[3]

Enormous changes have been inflicted on and instigated by man in the last four decades in Western society. The rapid technological and social change is exerting extreme pressure on humanity. To quote Alvin Toffler in *Future Shock*: 'There are discoverable limits to the amount of change that the human organism can absorb . . . by endlessly accelerating these limits, we may submit masses of men to demands they simply cannot tolerate'.[4] Life changes are a determining factor in stress-related illnesses. But the extent to which the events lead to ill health will depend to a large degree on a person's capacity to cope with stress.

The way an individual perceives a situation dramatically affects the stress response experienced. It is not so much the *actual* ability to cope with a situation that matters as the individual's *perception* of his ability to cope.

It is believed that up to 80 per cent of modern diseases have a stress-related background. These include hypertension, high blood pressure, coronary thrombosis, heart attack, migraine, hay fever and allergies, asthma, peptic ulcers, constipation, colitis, rheumatoid arthritis, menstrual difficulties, nervous dyspepsia, flatulence and indigestion, hyperthyroidism (overactive thyroid gland), diabetes mellitus, skin disorders, tuberculosis and depression.

We may not be able to alter the stress situations in life but we can alter how we cope. Natural healing techniques, relaxation techniques, meditation, diet and exercise can all help control or decrease the stress response and thereby lessen one's susceptibility to stress-related diseases.

CHAPTER THREE

Diet

*It's a very strange thing, as strange as strange can be
That whatever Miss T eats turns into Miss T.*

WALTER DE LA MARE

Diet – the word has connotations of deprivation. In the Oxford dictionary diet is defined as 'feed on special food as medical regimen or punishment'. This 'punishment' aspect causes most people to baulk at the mention of any diet, which is perceived as forced deprivation of all the tasty goodies that make eating pleasurable. This is a somewhat confused perception. Incorrect diet, although pleasurable to the palate, can be the direct cause of ill health, which can make life intolerably unpleasant, while correct diet can be the passport to fulfilment, health and longevity.

Few can honestly say they enjoy vibrant, boundless health, free from niggling aches, pains, allergies and mood swings. In place of the dynamic energy which is our birthright, we have been conditioned to accept health as simply the absence of disease. Western nations spend millions on caring for the sick, and thousands of man-hours are lost every year through minor illnesses and impaired performance. Much of this needless suffering and expense could be

alleviated if just a fraction of the money spent on remedial health care was channelled into education on diet, nutrition and prevention.

The one area of our lives over which most of us have total control is diet. It is also probably *the* most important factor in the maintenance of health and can be the greatest villain in the development of disease. The human body is constructed from the food we eat. Because we are constructed of energy fields, we are dependent on the energies we absorb from food. We should therefore eat foods compatible with our electrical energy needs that will stimulate rather than obstruct the free flow of energy in the body.

In the modern world an alarming amount of food is 'dead'. Pesticides, fertilizers, irradiation and chemical additives serve to deplete the natural energy in food thereby depriving us of the vitality required to construct a healthy body. The increasing pressures of modern life also cause disruptions in the energy flow. Vitamins, minerals, proteins, fats and carbohydrates are of no value if our bodies cannot assimilate them because they are out of balance, or if the food causes negative side-effects.

The value of plant energy is mentioned by world-renowned healer and psychic Edgar Cayce in the book *The Hidden Laws of the Earth*: 'Energy values in the food we eat are of great importance. Where does the energy in our food come from? The solar energy reaching the earth is absorbed by the leaves of plants. In the plants it joins with water, minerals and nitrogen compounds which the roots have sucked up from the ground and also carbonic acid, a gas which man breathes out as a waste product and which has been gathered by the plant from the air. The sun's energy is transferred into a new energy, and the plant grows, builds up its patterned structure, blooms and fruits. The energy becomes fixed in a state of rest and is then potential energy. In other words, chemical vital energy is produced by plants from solar energy. Man eats the plants and then utilises the chemical vital energy. Food from plants is higher in potential energy than that from animal products. Eating animal products is eating the energy second-hand.'[1]

We know energy circulates throughout the body, influencing all the organs and body parts. Organs rely on correct energy circulation for proper functioning. Insufficient or depleted energy could damage the organs and damaged organs will, in turn, interfere with the normal circulation of energy throughout the rest of the body.

One can equate this energy with a fire. Fire is vibrant, active and dynamic. In order to burn brightly, a fire needs high-quality wood. If anything interferes with the performance of the fire, for example low-quality wood, the fire may go out. The object is to build a strong, healthy fire to provide lasting heat, to ensure the fire is resilient and will therefore not be drastically affected by external factors. Low-quality wood burns badly and does not generate sufficient

heat, thus more wood is constantly required to feed the deficient flame.

Relating this to the body, if the vital energy symbolizes a fire, the wood can be equated with food. A body sustained on depleted junk food does not receive the necessary vitamins and minerals to function efficiently. As a result, the brain sends out messages for more nourishment. This craving is often dealt with by the consumption of caffeine, alchohol and sugar-laden drinks. This is the equivalent of putting petrol on the fire. A short sharp burst of instant energy is provided, but this is short-lived and suffers rapid burn-out. Then more 'petrol' is required to boost the flame again. This process cannot be maintained indefinitely without the body suffering for it. The fire needs to be sustained with the correct nourishment in order to burn steadily, strongly and continuously to create the energy necessary for a healthy body and mind.

Depleted or stimulating food and drink inflict stress on the body. Some form of reaction to this stress is inevitable. Physical manifestations will become apparent in the body systems, depending on where a person's particular weaknesses lie. Reactions often manifest via the endocrine system and could include asthma attacks, allergic reactions, palpitations, hyperventilation, and other disorders which can be directly or indirectly related to the adrenal glands. Reactions could also affect the thyroid, resulting in thyroid-related problems like depression and irritability.

In women these effects often accumulate in the uterus, to be released once a month as painful, heavy periods. If severe stress accumulates with no release, cysts and fibroids could develop in the ovaries and uterus. Modern medicine 'repairs' these problems with surgery. As the root of the problem – namely, incorrect fuel on the fire – is not dealt with, the stress will merely accumulate and resort to other outlets like the adrenal glands and thyroid. Young girls who suffer from allergies or asthma in childhood often grow out of them during puberty. This is because the body adjusts to release the stress via menstruation. Male reactions tend to be connected to adrenal output and can manifest as heart attacks, or be related to the thyroid and manifest in hair loss and metabolic disorders. In later life, if the internal climate is not corrected, men may suffer prostate problems.

Relating this to external stress factors, if the fire is well nourished and resilient, the body will deal more effectively with external stress. Emotional situations require more energy – thus the fire burns faster and more wood is required. If the fire is deficient, a stress situation will really take its toll. A strong fire may falter but will not suffer burn-out and will therefore enable one to handle a stress situation more effectively.

Nutrition is involved in every bodily activity and diet furnishes the raw materials or nutrients required for the synthesis of chemical substances indispensable to the body's growth, maintenance and repair. Unfortunately the modern trend is towards food empty of essential nutrients. Whatever happened to our natural instincts? Animals instinctively know which plants and grasses are good for them and which are bad, and will choose to eat those beneficial to their health and avoid those detrimental. We humans, however, are rather perverse – we have developed a tendency to eat food that is bad for us based purely on the sensuous taste and pleasure value. This tendency can be cited as one of the major causes of disease today.

Many health problems – heart disease, arthritis, kidney failure, gall bladder disorders, cancer and hyperactivity – can be related to incorrect diet. More disturbing and less frequently acknowledged are the mental complaints which may be related to improper nutrition.

The brain is extremely sensitive. When essential proteins, fatty acids, vitamins and minerals are not sufficiently available, brain cells degenerate rapidly causing a deteriorating emotional and intellectual state.[2] If food intake is inadequate the brain, like the body, must draw on reserves to function. Eventually the reserves are depleted and the person becomes stressed. If this continues, minor emotional symptoms can escalate into full-blown neuroses.

Deficient diet has been directly related to criminal behaviour, lowered IQ and aggressive tendencies. Excess consumption of three foods, artificial sugar, wheat and rye products, and meat, can be accompanied by aggressive behaviour. In the Western world, consumption of these products is exceptionally high, and this coincides with a preponderance of violent crimes.

Studies in the US have linked juvenile delinquency with low blood sugar, vitamin deficiencies, lead pollution and food allergies. In Britain, the British Society for Nutritional Medicine believes that teenage consumption of junk food and soft drinks is to blame for the rise in soccer hooliganism and other youthful violence. Crime in Britain is higher than at any other time in recent history.

Inadequate diet is also related to behavioural problems and learning difficulties in children. Bad eating habits can lead to everything from anaemia to low IQ. Children's IQ levels apparently drop if they consume quantities of refined foods.

Many types of food on the market today should be labelled 'toxic'. Refined carbohydrates are classified as 'susceptibility agents' (oversupply encourages disease). Since refined carbohydrates are grossly lacking in vitamins, minerals, essential fats and protein, these foodstuffs are quite correctly labelled 'empty calories'. This group embraces table sugar, many precooked breakfast cereals, white flour, white (polished) rice, all highly sweetened foods (desserts, sweetened beverages, etc.) and both sweetened and unsweetened baked goods made from white wheat flour.

Apart from refined food we are also subjected to gross chemical contamination, which is harmful and can cause multiple sensitivities amongst other things. Contamination occurs in two main areas: the first is herbicide, pesticide or weedkiller residues on fruit and vegetables and the presence of traces of synthetic hormones and antibiotics in meat. The second is the addition of chemicals to foods in order to improve their appearance and therefore saleability. The quantities of chemicals consumed are horrifying.

In one year the average person breathes in 2 grams of solid pollution, eats 12lbs of food additives, has a gallon of herbicides and pesticides sprayed on the fruits and vegetables they eat, and receives nitrates, hormones and antibotic residues from both water and food. No less than 6000 new chemicals have been introduced into our food, our homes and the world around us in the last decade. Although we are equipped with clever mechanisms for detoxifying harmful substances, for many of us those mechanisms are becoming overloaded. When the total body burden of pollutants exceeds our ability to detoxify, these substances are integrated into bone, fat, brain and other tissues. The effects of pollution are cumulative.[3]

The list of additives in ice-cream sounds like a science project. Many nutritionists now refer to ice-cream as 'the garbage dump food'. These are some additives found in commercially produced ice-cream:

Piperonal – used in place of vanilla – is a chemical used to treat lice

Diethyl glucol – a cheap chemical used as an emulsifier instead of eggs – is used in antifreeze and paint removers

Butyraldehyde – used in nut-flavoured ice-cream – one of the ingredients in rubber cement

Amyl acetate – used for banana flavour – is also an oil paint solvent

Ethyl acetate – used for pineapple flavour – also used as a cleaner for leather and textiles

Aldehyde C17 – flavours cherry ice-cream – an inflammable liquid used in aniline dyes, plastic and rubber.

The additivies in many modern foods combine to form a lethal cocktail. Man is not designed to consume inorganic foodstuffs and the increased consumption of chemical compounds leaves toxic waste in the cells. If we continue at this rate we will soon be positively non-biodegradable. In fact rumour has it that, due to chemical residue, a human corpse now takes longer to decompose.

Food processing has two major effects. First, it often changes and reverses the sodium/potassium ratio in foods. In the natural state most fruits and vegetables contain high levels of potassium and low levels of sodium. The body is good at conserving sodium and therefore requires very little; in contrast it is bad at conserving potassium and loses this vital element with alarming ease. Therefore a high potassium and low sodium diet is necessary. Another major effect of food processing is a reduction in the vitamin content of food, in some cases by a factor of ten times and in most cases by at least half. It is therefore possible to become vitamin deficient in the midst of plenty.[4]

Diseases associated with high levels of pollutants include all forms of arthritis, allergies, candidiasis, ME, repeated infections, hyperactivity, high blood pressure, asthma, acne, eczema and schizophrenia. Minor symptoms associated with an increased body burden of pollutants include lethargy, drowsiness, mood swings, inability to concentrate, intolerance of fat or alchohol, poor skin, body odour, headaches, nausea, skin rashes, frequent infections and multiple allergies. All of these symptoms can occur for other reasons as well, but they are far more likely to occur in those who are not adequately nourished.[5]

There is no adage as accurate as 'you are what you eat'. A healthy, balanced diet rich in natural organic foods will build a strong, healthy, disease-resistant body and mind, while a diet loaded with sugar, meat and chemically treated 'dead' food will not only create the perfect breeding ground for disease, it may also drive you crazy!

THE ART OF REFLEXOLOGY

He shall subdue the people under us:
and the nations under our feet.

PSALMS 47:3

THE human foot is an architectural master-piece. This delicate structure, but a fraction of the size of the body, balances, supports and transports the entire body weight. The ease with which these relatively small appendages adapt to their task is nothing short of astounding. Few people pay much attention to their feet, which take a severe beating on their path through life. Little notice is given to the serious health damage caused by self-induced foot disorders – disorders which inevitably cause problems elsewhere in the body. This can occur on two levels.

Firstly, the structure of the foot forms our base and foundation. A strong foundation relies on correct alignment and joint function and any impairment to the functions will displace the centre of gravity. Other areas of the body will then overcompensate causing knee, leg and calf pain as well as back problems. Poor circulation, incorrect posture, sore backs and headaches can be attributed to tired, aching feet and swollen ankles. The structure of the foot can be severely damaged by ill-fitting shoes, walking incorrectly, and any other form of excessive stress, like running and ballet. These conditions cause foot deformities ranging from corns and calluses to more serious damage like bunions and enlarged toe joints.

Foot deformities and irregularities also affect the reflexes and meridians on which they manifest. This can, in turn, affect the corresponding body parts by causing congestion in energy flow, and possibly affecting associated organs.

To a reflexologist, feet tell a thousand stories. The foot represents the body and every nick and crevice holds a key to the nature of the problem. A professional, responsible and successful practitioner will have a thorough knowledge of foot structure, reflexes and meridians.

ANATOMY OF THE FOOT

The average foot contains 26 small bones, 2 sesamoids (smaller bones), 114 ligaments and 20 muscles. These are joined together with connective tissue, blood vessels and nerves and covered in layers of skin. This finely tuned, intricate structure is balanced on two main arches – one, from the heel to the base of the little toe, the other from heel to big toe.

The hands and feet contain the same number of bones – together they make up half the bones of the body. In each foot are fourteen phalanges – toe bones. There are three phalanges in each toe, except the big toe which contains two. These are joined by ligaments to the five metatarsals – long bones that extend the length of the foot towards the heel.

The midfoot is constructed of three cuneiform bones. These help stabilize and support body weight. The longitudinal/transverse arch, which extends from the heel to the ball of the foot, is built of the navicular, cuboid and cuneiform bones.

The heel – calcaneus – bears the brunt of our weight. It is therefore insulated with protective layers of fat to cushion the impact of each footstep. The talus – ankle bone – provides up and down leverage. The joints, muscles and tendons control the motions of the foot.

It is obvious the foot is a marvellously constructed mechanism. Lamentably, insufficient attention is paid to the feet considering their impressive role in our lives. The common phrase, 'My feet are killing me', could be answered with, 'You are killing your feet'. Reflexology recognizes the vital role of feet in health and healing, and aims to emphasize that if you take care of your feet, they will take care of you.

VERTICAL/LONGITUDINAL ZONES

Zone Therapy as developed by Dr W. Fitzgerald can be useful for 'mapping' areas of the body reflected on the feet. According to Fitzgerald,

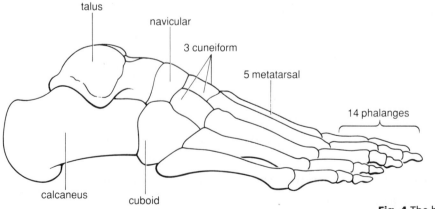

talus
navicular
3 cuneiform
5 metatarsal
14 phalanges
calcaneus
cuboid

Fig. 4 The bones of the foot

ten equal longitudinal zones run the length of the body from the head down to the toes, as well as from the head to the fingers. These zones are calculated from a central line through the body which runs parallel to the spine. Each foot represents half of the body, and each toe, a zone. The spine is the dividing line and the zones radiate outwards, numbered one to five each way. Half the spine is represented on the instep of each foot. All organs on the right side of the body are represented on the right foot; those on the left of the body on the left foot. An organ or gland found in a specific zone has its reflex in the corresponding zone of the foot.

ZONES VERSUS MERIDIANS

Most reflexologists accept the concept of body congestions being reflected in the zones described by Fitzgerald. To quote Kevin and Barbara Kunz from their book, *The Complete Guide to Foot Reflexology*: 'Sometimes when a medical diagnosis has not been possible a "generalised" pain somewhere in the body can be traced, using the zones, to a "distinct" area of the foot. As a practice exercise, look at the illustration. Look at the spot marked "x" where, let's say, there's some pain or injury. By tracing along the appropriate zone down into the foot, you can find sensitivity there too. Since the basic principle of reflexology is that build-up will occur in that zone of the foot as a result of the stress or injury in spot "x", the zonal relationships provide guidelines for locating pain more precisely.'

This I disagree with. No definite proof supports this zone theory. To my mind the zones should only be used as a *guideline* for mapping the body on to the feet – not as a complete mirror image. I consider that the concept of zones in the hands is not relevant as I would see the hands falling into zone 5 and not as divided into ten separate zones.

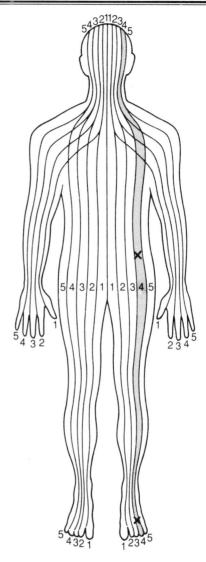

Fig. 5

I believe reflexology originally developed in conjunction with acupuncture. The reason for massaging the foot was primarily to stimulate the six main meridians that run through the feet. During the course of history, the relationship between these two practices was somehow lost and forgotten. When reflexology re-emerged in the West, researchers and practitioners came to the conclusion that stimulating the feet caused a reaction in the body, but were not sure how this was actuated. As the Eastern meridian knowledge had not arrived in the West at that stage, the relationship with the meridians was not realized, so the zone theory was born.

There are parallels between the meridians and zones. Take, for example, the relationship between the eyes and the kidneys. In zone theory, problems with the eyes can be related to kidney disorders as both fall into zone 2. This relationship also occurs in the meridians. The bladder meridian begins at the eyes, as does the stomach meridian. The stomach meridian penetrates the kidneys and imbalances may manifest as dark shadows or puffiness under the eyes. Orthodox medicine, too, accepts these signs as being indicative of kidney disorders. The stomach meridian ends in the second toe, with an internal branch of the same meridian in the third toe. Here we have the connection with the toes – the second and third toes represent the eye reflexes *and* the stomach meridian.

Before we proceed with the detailed mapping of the feet, I want to propose a new way to approach this, which works in conjunction with the meridians and their pathways. Careful study of the meridian pathways and related organs will clarify organ location on reflexology charts and explain how organ reflexes relate to the meridians. Meridians are not straight lines – zones are. Meridians have curved, and sometimes zig-zag, pathways that traverse throughout the body including the feet. Thus, the sections of the meridians found in the torso, and therefore the related organs, are what should be mirrored on to the foot and the reflexes.

To establish how reflexes, meridians and organs are connected, look first at the toes. The second and third toes correspond to the eye reflexes, the fourth and fifth toes to the ear reflexes. The tips of all the toes represent the sinus reflexes. When relating meridians to the

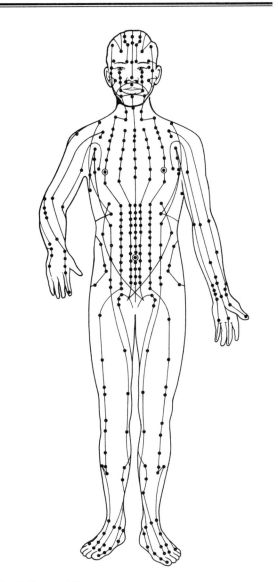

Fig. 6 The meridians

situation of the reflexes, parallels can be drawn.

The most relevant meridian is the stomach meridian. This has its origin under the eyes, lateral to the nose. It has a descending pathway which ends in the second toe – the eye reflex. One of the internal branches ends in the third toe – also the eye reflex. Another branch ends in the first toe affecting the nose reflex. As the

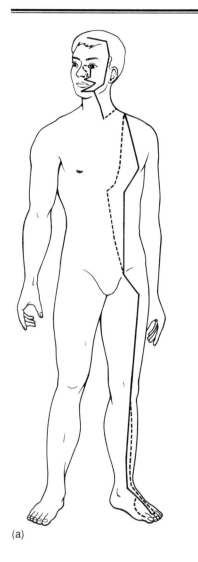

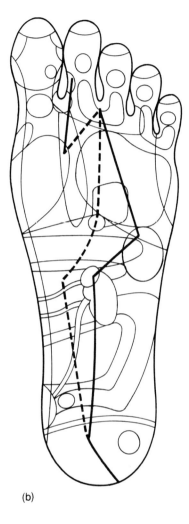

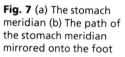

Fig. 7 (a) The stomach meridian (b) The path of the stomach meridian mirrored onto the foot

(a)   (b)

sinus reflexes are situated on the tips of all the toes, sinuses are affected by the toes, as is the facial section of the stomach meridian which is also represented in the toes. The curved path of the stomach meridian affects the sinuses, throat, lungs, diaphragm, spleen, liver, gall bladder, stomach, pancreas, duodenum, adrenal glands, kidneys, large intestine, small intestine and pelvic region. All the reflexes of these organs are situated under the second and third toes, except the spleen reflex, which is situated

mainly under the fourth toe. The zig-zag pathway of the meridian is evident on the torso as well as the feet.

The gall bladder meridian begins in the face next to the eyes and descends to end in the fourth toe. It circulates around the ear, and therefore directly relates to the ear reflex which is situated on the fourth toe. The internal branch meridian is represented in the big toe (towards the second toe), which relates to the mastoid and Eustachian tube reflexes – linking

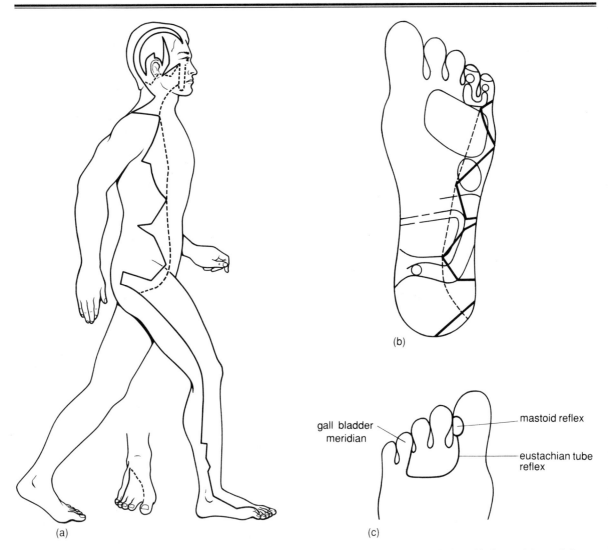

gall bladder
meridian

mastoid reflex

eustachian tube
reflex

(a)

(b)

(c)

Fig. 8 (a) The gall bladder meridian (b) The gall bladder meridian mirrored on to the left foot (c) the positions of the mastoid and Eustachian tube reflexes

the first toe to the fourth toe. The gall bladder meridian penetrates the lungs, liver, gall bladder, spleen, large intestine and hip area. According to reflexology charts the reflexes for a part of all these organs are situated below the fourth toe, and to the outer side of the foot.

The liver and spleen/pancreas meridians both begin in the big toe and end in the breast region. Both meridians have internal branches which

run through the throat area, and therefore indirectly affect the throat and thyroid. (Figure 9.) The thyroid is also affected by the stomach meridian, as mentioned. Bunions are usually situated on the spleen/pancreas meridian and around the thyroid reflex, and therefore affect the thyroid as well. Some reflexologists find the thyroid is 'helped' when reflexes on the second toe and around the big toe are worked on. These

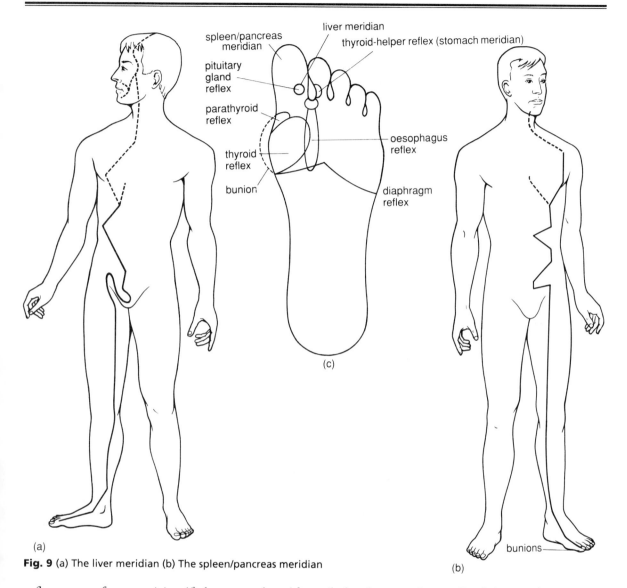

Fig. 9 (a) The liver meridian (b) The spleen/pancreas meridian

reflexes are often sensitive if there are thyroid disorders. This is again due to stimulating the meridians. (Figure 9c.)

The thyroid reflex has recently been repositioned by some reflexologists, to the area near the big toe – the neck area (see Figure 10). This is probably because in this position it fits in more accurately with the 'image' of the body stipulated in zone therapy. However, most charts and books have retained this as a thyroid 'helper' area as they realized that working on the 'old' reflex area (on the ball of the foot, directly below the big toe) was effective in alleviating thyroid complaints.

According to all reflexology charts, the big toe incorporates the head and brain reflexes. Two important glands – namely the pituitary and pineal glands – are situated in the brain, so their reflexes would be found in the brain reflex area of the big toe. Relating this to meridians – the

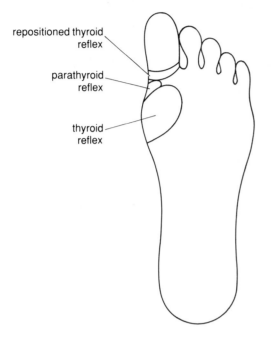

repositioned thyroid reflex

parathyroid reflex

thyroid reflex

Fig. 10 The position of the thyroid reflex

pituitary gland is situated on the liver meridian, the internal branch of which runs through the neck as well as the head. (See Figure 9.)

Note the position of the uterus/prostate reflexes between the heel and ankle bone on the inside of the foot. The main reason why this area is effective in complaints relating to the uterus and prostate is the presence of the kidney meridian. The kidney meridian also penetrates the uterus/prostate in the body, and according to Chinese medicine the kidneys store the 'Jing' – a vital essence involved in reproduction. The kidney meridian also exerts an indirect effect on these organs via the internal branch meridian which runs through the lumbar vertebrae. The nerves from the lumbar vertebrae supply the organs mentioned. It is therefore understandable why many women suffer back problems during menstruation and when giving birth.

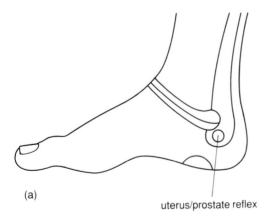

(a)

uterus/prostate reflex

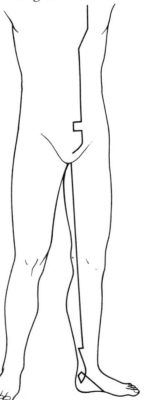

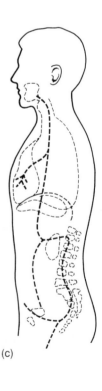

(b)

(c)

Fig. 11 (a) The position of the uterus/prostrate reflex (b) Section of the kidney meridian (c) Internal branch of the kidney meridian running through the lumbar vertebrae

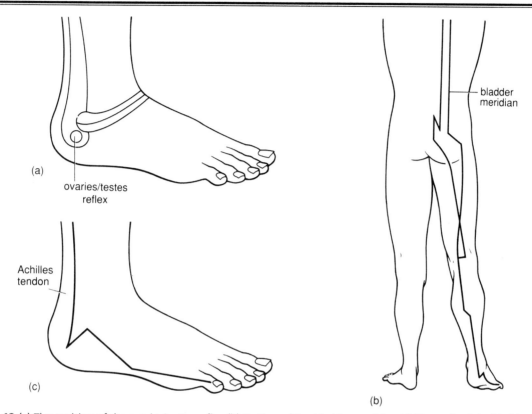

Fig. 12 (a) The position of the ovaries/testes reflex (b) Section of the bladder meridian (c) The path of the bladder meridian on the foot

The reflexes for the ovaries/testes are situated between the heel and ankle bone on the outside of the foot. The bladder meridian runs through this area of the foot influencing these reflexes. In the body, the bladder meridian also runs through the lumbar vertebrae, and, as with the kidneys, the nerve supply affects these organs. On many charts, reflexes for chronic sciatica, uterus, prostate and rectum (anus) are situated on both sides of the Achilles tendon. As this area incorporates the kidney and bladder meridians, stimulation here affects everything along these meridian paths, including the organs just mentioned.

The heart reflex has been repositioned on many new charts, to the area where I have placed the thyroid reflex – again, probably to fit in with zone therapy mapping. Prior to its repositioning, the heart reflex was placed where I describe it. Apart from the uterus/prostate and other organs, the kidney meridian also passes through the solar plexus and the heart, almost parallel to the stomach meridian on the inner side of the breast region. This is the only meridian that passes through the solar plexus. This part of the meridian, plus one of its small branches, when mirrored on to the feet overlap at one point – on the actual heart meridian. The kidney meridian starts in the foot at the solar plexus reflex. The heart reflex, though slightly up to one side, touches the solar plexus reflex. One of the internal branches starts from the little toe, runs across the sole of the upper foot and ends at the solar plexus reflex. It penetrates the heart reflex. In the body, a small internal branch also penetrates the heart.

To take this concept of mapping the feet a

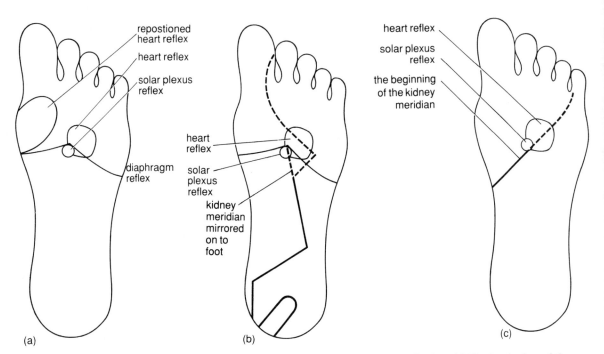

Fig. 13 (a) The position of the heart reflex (b) The kidney meridian mirrored on to the foot (c) The beginning of the kidney meridian

step further, take note of the sciatic nerve, which is mapped as a reflex in a band running horizontally across the heel. This is not only a reflex. Part of the actual nerve is situated in the heel. It often happens that massage to this area relieves sciatic problems. This is because the bladder meridian runs along the same pathway as the sciatic nerve, and massage here stimulates both the bladder meridian and the sciatic nerve.

The band across the top of the ankle, from inner to outer ankle bones, represents reflexes for the groin lymph system. All six meridians located in the feet run through the pelvic region, so problems here can be traced to a specific area and meridian.

The bladder meridian is the only meridian that runs along the spine, and therefore has a profound effect on the spinal cord and nerves. It is the longest meridian in the body, touches all

the vertebrae and enters the brain. It therefore affects the central nervous system and, via the nerve supply, indirectly affects all the organs in the body.

Two extra meridians, referred to as 'vessel' meridians, should also be mentioned. The Governing vessel runs along the spinal cord at the back of the body, the Conception vessel runs midline along the front of the body, thus forming a circuit. This is clearly depicted if the foot is mirrored on to a side-view of the body showing these meridians (Figure 15).

The meridians situated in the arms do not penetrate any major organs as they run from face to fingers or vice versa.

It is thus obvious that the reflexes on the feet are closely related to the meridian pathways, and this indicates why study of meridians should be incorporated with reflexology.

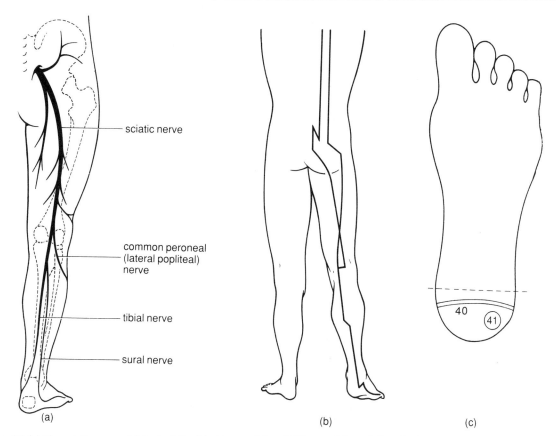

Fig. 14 (a) The sciatic nerve (b) Part of the bladder meridian (c) The position of the sciatic nerve and pelvis reflexes

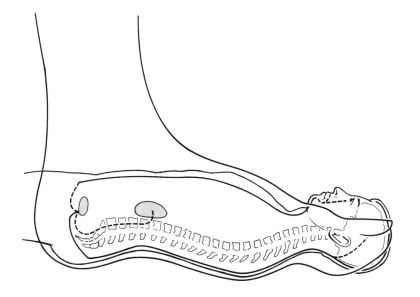

Fig. 15 The foot mirrored of the body showing the governing vessel which runs along the spinal cord and the conception vessel which runs along the front of the body

Mapping the Feet

*The head and feet keep warm
The rest will take no harm*
ANONYMOUS

Understanding the structure of the feet in relation to the body is the first and most important step to understanding reflexology. It is, in fact, very simple, as the feet are a microcosm or mini-map of the whole body and all the organs and body parts are reflected on the feet in a similar arrangement as in the body. These reflexes are found on the soles, tops and along the inside and outside of the feet and their positions follow a logical anatomical pattern.

MAPPING THE REFLEXES ON THE FEET

The body itself is divided horizontally into four parts: the head and neck area; the thoracic area from the shoulders to the diaphragm; the abdominal area from the diaphragm to the pelvic area; and the pelvis. These areas can be clearly delineated on the feet and provide a precise picture of the body as it is reflected on the feet. We will therefore examine the situation of body organs in horizontal divisions as this facilitates easy study and reference, and it also fits in more accurately with the massage technique I teach. This is easier to understand if studied together with the meridians.

The sections described above are also clearly visible in the foot structure: the head and neck area = the toes; the thoracic area = the ball of the foot; the abdominal area = the arch; the pelvic area = the heel. Also, the reproductive area = the ankle; the spine = the inner foot; the outer body = the outer foot; circulation and breasts = tops of the feet.

THE HEAD AND NECK AREA – THE TOES

The toes incorporate reflexes to all parts of the body found above the shoulder girdle. If you imagine the two big toes as two half heads with a common neck the positions of the reflexes are placed very logically. Obviously some reflexes overlap as they do in the body. Each big toe contains reflex points for the pituitary gland,

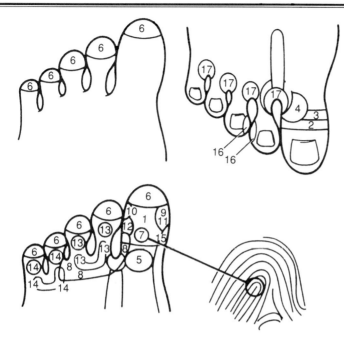

1. brain
2. mouth
3. nose
4. tonsils
5. neck
6. sinus, teeth and top of head
7. pituitary gland
8. eustachian tube
9. pineal gland
10. temples
11. hypothalamus
12. mastoid
13. eyes
14. ears
15. cervical spine (C1–C7)
16. lachrymal glands (tearducts)
17. upper lymph system
18. speech centre

Fig. 16 The head and neck area

pineal gland, hypothalamus, brain, temples, teeth, the seven cervical (neck) vertebrae, sinuses, mastoid, tonsils, nose, mouth and other face reflexes as well as part of the Eustachian tubes.

The other four toes on each foot contain reflex points for the eyes, ears, teeth, sinuses, lachrymal glands (tearducts), speech centre, upper lymph system, collar bone (shoulder girdle), Eustachian tubes, chronic eyes and ears.

The Head and the Brain

Reflexes of the head and the brain are on the pads of the big toes from the tip behind the nail down over the metatarsal bone; reflexes for the sides of the head and brain are on the sides of the big toes. On the top of the toes are the face reflexes including the mouth, nose, teeth and tonsils. At the base of the big toe are the neck reflexes.

Sinuses

The sinuses are cavities within the skull bones situated above and to the sides of the nose, in the cheekbones and behind the eyebrows. They communicate with the nasal cavities through small openings. They act as protection for the eyes and the brain and give resonance to the voice.

The reflexes are situated on the tips of all the toes.

The Pituitary Gland

This gland, known also as the 'master gland', is considered the most important in the body as it controls the functions of all the endocrine glands. About the size and shape of a cherry, the pituitary gland is attached to the base of the brain. Numerous hormones are produced by this gland – these influence growth, sexual development, metabolism, pregnancy, mineral and sugar content of the blood, fluid retention and energy levels.

The reflex point is found on both feet where the whorl of the toe print converges into a central point. It is usually situated on the inner side of the toe and often requires a little searching. More often than not, this reflex is found to be off-centre. Since the hormonal system is extremely sensitive and easily thrown off-balance, this reflex is usually very tender.

The Hypothalamus

A number of bodily activities are controlled by this part of the brain. It regulates the autonomic nervous system and controls emotional reactions, appetite, body temperature and sleep.

The hypothalamus reflex areas are found on both feet on the outer side and top of the big toe – the same reflex point as the pineal gland.

The Pineal Gland

The pineal gland is a small gland situated within the hypothalamus section of the brain. Its functions are not completely understood but it is known to stimulate the cells in the skin to produce the black pigment melanin. It is thought to play a part in mood and circadian rhythms, and is sometimes referred to as the psychic 'third eye'.

The reflexes are on both feet on the outer tip of the big toes – the same as the hypothalamus reflex.

The Teeth

The reflexes to the teeth are exactly distributed over the ten toes: incisors on the big toe; incisors and canine teeth on the second toe; premolars on the third toe; molars on the fourth toe; wisdom teeth on the fifth toe. These reflexes are in the same position as the sinus reflexes.

The Eyes

The eyes are important sensory organs – the organs of sight. The nerve tissue of the retina receives impressions of images via the pupils and the lens. From this the optic nerve conveys the impressions to the visual area of the cerebral cortex where they are interpreted.

These reflexes are on both feet on the cush-ions of the second and third toes and may extend slightly down the toes. Reflexes for chronic eye conditions are on the 'shelf' at the base of these two toes.

The Ears

The ear is the organ of hearing. It is a highly complex system of cavities, bones and membranes, constructed in such a way that sound waves in the atmosphere are caught up and transmitted to the hearing centre in the temporal lobe of the cerebral cortex. The ear also plays a part in maintaining balance.

The reflexes are situated on both feet on the cushions of the fourth and fifth toes and may extend slightly down the toes. The reflexes for the Eustachian tubes extend from the inner side of the big toe along the base of the second and third toes to the fourth toe. Reflexes for chronic ear conditions are found on the 'shelf' at the base of these two toes – the same section as the Eustachian tubes. The mastoid – the part of the skull behind the ear which contains the air spaces that communicate with the ear – is also treated on these reflexes.

The Tonsils

These are paired organs composed of lymphatic tissue and thought to be involved in defence of the throat area.

The reflexes are found on both feet – on the top of the foot at the base of the big toe near the web between the big and second toes.

The Lymphatic System

The lymphatic system is a network of lymphatic vessels situated throughout the body which drain tissue fluid surrounding the cells in the body. Lymph nodes filter the lymph to prevent infection passing into the bloodstream and add lymphocytes which are important for the formation of antibodies and immunological

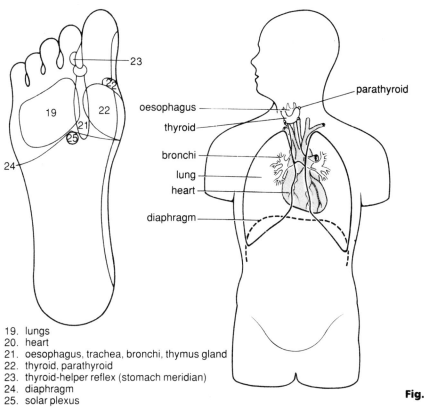
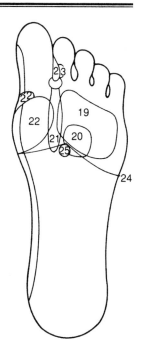

oesophagus
thyroid
bronchi
lung
heart
diaphragm

parathyroid

19. lungs
20. heart
21. oesophagus, trachea, bronchi, thymus gland
22. thyroid, parathyroid
23. thyroid-helper reflex (stomach meridian)
24. diaphragm
25. solar plexus

Fig. 17 The thoracic area

reactions. The main sites of the lymph nodes are in the neck, armpit, breast, abdomen, groin, pelvis and behind the knee.

On the front of the foot, the webs between the toes are the reflexes for lymph drainage in the neck and chest region of the body. Lymph reflexes for the groin area are linked to the reproductive system and found in the same area as the reflexes for the Fallopian tubes and vas deferens described later in this chapter. These reflexes run across the top of the foot from the inner ankle bone to the outer ankle bone and incorporate the six main meridians. Congestions in the groin can be traced to a specific meridian and its organ depending on where these are situated.

THE THORACIC AREA – THE BALL OF THE FOOT

This section of the foot corresponds with the thoracic area in the body from the shoulder girdle to the diaphragm. Several vital reflexes are situated here: the heart, lungs, oesophagus, trachea, bronchi, thyroid and thymus glands, diaphragm and solar plexus.

The Lungs

The lungs are cone-shaped, spongy organs which lie in the thorax on either side of the heart. It is here that the process of respiration takes place – the exchange of oxygen for carbon dioxide. The air passages of the respiratory system found in the thorax are the trachea (windpipe) which divides into the bronchi to enter the left and right lungs.

The lung reflexes are found on the soles of both feet from the second toe (stomach meridian) to just past the fourth toe (gall bladder meridian). Reflexes of the trachea and bronchi are found below the big toe and second toes (stomach and liver meridians) connected to the lung reflex. These same reflexes are also found in similar positions on the tops of the feet.

The Heart

The heart is a hollow, cone-shaped, muscular organ which lies in the chest on the left side of the body in a space between the lungs. It acts as a pump circulating blood throughout the body. Efficient functioning of the heart is essential to allow good blood circulation, which is necessary for efficient transport of gases, foods and waste products. The chest area also contains other major vessels leading to and from the heart – the arteries, veins, vena cavae and aorta.

The reflex to the heart is situated on the sole of the left foot only – on the kidney meridian above the diaphragm level.

The Thymus Gland, Oesophagus, Trachea and Bronchi

The thymus gland is situated in the thoracic cavity. It is quite large in childhood, reaches maximum size at 10 to 12 years, then slowly regresses and almost disappears in adult life. It is involved in the immune system, but its only known function is the formation of lymphocytes.

The oesophagus is the gullet – a muscular tube passing from the pharynx down through the chest, and joining the stomach below the diaphragm. Food and fluid are propelled through it by peristalsis, the wave-like contractions of the intestinal walls.

The trachea is the windpipe. It passes down from the larynx into the chest where it divides into two bronchi, the main divisions of the trachea which enter the lungs.

All these reflexes are found on both feet in the same area – on the soles of the feet in a vertical band between the first and second toes.

The Thyroid Gland

The thyroid gland is located in the neck. It controls the rate of metabolism and maintains the correct amount of calcium in the blood.

This reflex is situated on both feet at the base of the big toe, down around the ball and into the groove below the bone. The most important part is the section along the bone. There is also a 'helper' reflex on the second toe – the stomach meridian.

The Parathyroid Glands

These are four small glands situated around the thyroid gland. Their main function is to maintain the correct amount of calcium and phosphorus in the blood and bones.

The reflex is situated on both feet at the base of the big toe on the outer side.

The Diaphragm

The diaphragm, one of the muscles of respiration, is a large, dome-shaped wall which separates the thorax from the abdomen. It is the most important muscle for breathing.

This reflex is situated on the soles of both feet, extends across all six meridians at the base of the ball of the foot separating the ball from the arch.

The Solar Plexus

The solar plexus is a network of sympathetic nerve ganglia in the abdomen and is the nerve supply to the abdominal organs below the diaphragm. It is sometimes referred to as the 'abdominal brain' or the 'nerve switchboard' and is situated behind the stomach and in front of the diaphragm.

The reflex is at the same level as the reflex to the diaphragm, located at a specific point in the centre of the diaphragm reflex. This point is visible on the foot as the apex of the arch that runs across the base of the ball of the foot. This reflex is most useful for inducing a relaxed state. It can relieve stress and nervousness, aid deep regular breathing and restore calm.

THE ABDOMINAL AREA – THE ARCH OF THE FOOT

The arch of the foot is clearly visible on the sole – the raised area which extends from the base of the ball to the beginning of the heel. It is divided into two parts: the upper part corresponds to the section of the body from the diaphragm to the waistline; the lower part corresponds to the section of the body from the waistline to the pelvic area.

Reflexes above the waistline: liver, gall bladder, stomach, pancreas, duodenum, spleen, adrenals and kidneys.

The Liver

The liver is the largest and most complex organ/gland in the body. It controls many of the chemical processes and has many functions. These include: processing nutrients from the blood; storing fats and proteins until the body needs them; detoxifying the blood and manufacturing bile for fat digestion; storing sugars in the form of glycogen to be used when the body needs an increased supply of energy.

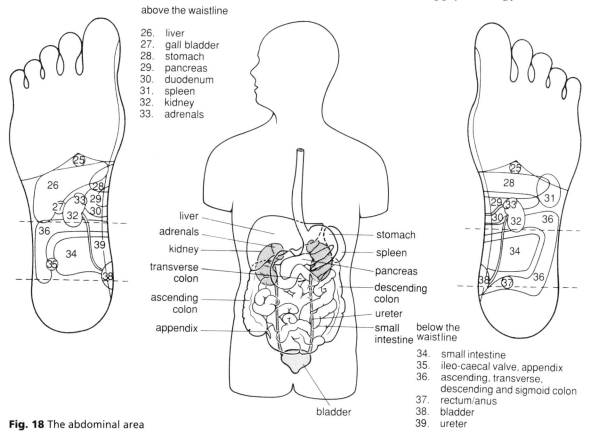

above the waistline

26. liver
27. gall bladder
28. stomach
29. pancreas
30. duodenum
31. spleen
32. kidney
33. adrenals

liver
adrenals
kidney
transverse colon
ascending colon
appendix

stomach
spleen
pancreas
descending colon
ureter
small intestine

bladder

below the waistline

34. small intestine
35. ileo-caecal valve, appendix
36. ascending, transverse, descending and sigmoid colon
37. rectum/anus
38. bladder
39. ureter

Fig. 18 The abdominal area

This reflex is found on the sole of the right foot only, below the diaphragm level, extending from the spleen/pancreas meridian on the inside of the foot to below the little toe. It ends just above the waistline.

The Gall Bladder

This is a small, muscular, pear-shaped sac attached to the under-surface of the liver. Its function is to excrete bile for food digestion.

The gall bladder reflex is on the sole of the right foot only, embedded within the liver reflex, beneath and between the third and fourth toes.

The Stomach

The stomach is a large, muscular sac which lies below the diaphragm mainly to the left side of the body. Food passes from the mouth down the oesophagus into the stomach where it is churned up and mixed with gastric juices and enzymes to start the digestive process.

The reflexes are found on the soles of both feet – extending from the big toe to the second toe on the right foot and the big toe to the outer edge of the fourth toe on the left foot. Horizontally, they are situated just below the diaphragm level.

The Pancreas

The pancreas is a large glandular structure in the abdomen. It is probably best known for the production of the hormones insulin and glucagon which are important in the control of sugar metabolism.

The reflexes are situated on the soles of both feet – more on the left foot than the right foot – below the stomach and above the waistline. On the right foot it extends to just below the big toe, and on the left foot as far as the fourth toe.

The Duodenum

This is the first, C-shaped part of the small intestine, about 20 to 25 centimetres long. It extends from the pyloric sphincter of the stomach to the jejunum. Pancreatic and common bile ducts open into it, releasing secretions responsible for the breakdown of food.

The reflexes are on the soles of both feet immediately below the pancreas, touching the waistline and extending inwards to the second toe.

The Spleen

The spleen is a large, very vascular, gland-like but ductless organ found on the left side of the body behind the stomach. It plays an important part in the immune system, and is part of the lymphatic system. It contains lymphatic tissue which manufactures the white blood cells, breaks down old red blood corpuscles and filters the lymph of toxins.

The reflex is found on the outer side of the left foot (opposite the liver reflex on the right foot), beneath the fourth toe (gall bladder meridian) just below the diaphragm, in line with the stomach reflex.

The Kidneys

The kidneys are part of the main excretory system of the body – the urinary system – which collectively refers to the kidneys, ureter tubes, urethra and bladder. They are two bean-shaped organs which filter toxins from the blood, produce urine and regulate the retention of important minerals and water.

The reflexes are found on the soles of both feet, positioned just above the waistline on the kidney and stomach meridians, just below the stomach reflex. The right kidney is positioned slightly lower than the left kidney.

The Adrenal Glands

These are two triangular endocrine glands situated on the upper tip of each kidney. As part of the endocrine system they perform numerous vital functions. The adrenal glands are divided into two distinct regions, the cortex and medulla. The adrenal cortex produces steroid hormones which regulate carbohydrate metabolism and have anti-allergic and anti-inflammatory properties. The cortex also produces hormones which control the reabsorption of sodium and water in the kidneys, as well as the secretion of potassium and the sex hormones testosterone, oestrogen and progesterone. The adrenal medulla produces adrenaline and noradrenaline which work in conjunction with the sympathetic nervous system. The output of adrenaline is increased at times of anxiety and stress and is responsible for organ changes in the 'fight-or-flight' situation. The reflexes are situated on the soles of both feet on top of the kidney reflexes.

Reflexes below the waistline: small intestine, ileo-caecal valve, appendix, large intestine, adrenals, kidneys, ureters, bladder.

The Small Intestine

This is a muscular tube about 6 to 7 metres in length and is the main area of the digestive tract where absorption takes place. It leads from the pyloric sphincter of the stomach to the caecum of the large intestine and lies in a coiled position in the abdominal cavity surrounded by the large intestine. The small intestine is divided into three sections – the duodenum, jejunum and the ileum.

The reflex is situated on the soles of both feet, under the large intestine reflex, extending horizontally across the arch to below the fourth toe.

The Ileo-Caecal Valve

This valve is situated where the small intestine and large intestine join, and therefore controls the passage of contents of the small intestine through to the large intestine. It prevents back-flow of faecal matter from the large intestine and controls mucous secretions.

The reflex is found on the sole of the right foot below and between the third and fourth toes, just above the level of the pelvic floor.

The Appendix

The appendix is a worm-like tube about 9 to 10 centimetres in length, with a blind end projecting downwards from the caecum of the large intestine in the lower right part of the abdominal cavity. Located directly below the ileo-caecal valve, it helps lubricate the large intestine, is rich in lymphoid tissue and secretes anti-bodies.

The reflex is situated on the sole of the right foot only, in the same area as the ileo-caecal valve.

The Large Intestine

This is a tube about 1.5 metres in length which surrounds the small intestine. It starts on the right side of the body at the caecum (ileo-caecal valve), goes up the right side to below the liver where it bends to the left (hepatic flexure) and passes across the abdomen as the transverse colon. At the left side of the abdomen, it bends down below the spleen (splenic flexure) to become the descending colon which passes down the left side of the abdomen. It then turns towards the midline and takes the shape of a double S-shaped bend known as the sigmoid flexure. This leads into the rectum which in turn becomes the anus.

When the residue of food reaches the large intestine it is in fluid form. The function of the large intestine is to remove some of the water and salts by absorption and to convert the waste matter into faeces ready for excretion.

The reflexes are found on the soles of both feet. On the right foot this begins just below the reflex for the ileo-caecal valve and extends upwards (ascending colon), turns just below the liver reflex to become the transverse colon which extends across the entire foot. It continues across to the left foot and turns just below the spleen reflex to become the descending colon. Just above the pelvic floor it turns again into the sigmoid colon which ends at the reflex of the rectum/anus.

The Ureters

The ureters are muscular tubes about 30 centimetres in length, which connect the kidneys and bladder and function as a passageway for urine. There are two tubes, one from each kid-ney, which pass downward through the abdomen into the pelvis where they enter the bladder.

The reflexes are situated on the soles of both feet linking the kidney reflexes to the bladder reflexes, which are situated on the inner side of the instep. The ureter reflexes can often be seen as distinct lines running down the arch.

The Bladder

The bladder is an elastic muscular sac situated in the centre of the pelvis. Urine for excretion passes from the kidneys down the ureters and is stored in the bladder until it is eliminated via the urethra.

The reflexes are found on both feet, on the side of the foot below the inner ankle bone on the heel line. This reflex is often clearly visible as a puffy area.

THE PELVIC AREA – THE HEEL OF THE FOOT

Few organs are represented here, but this area is of vital importance as all six main meridians

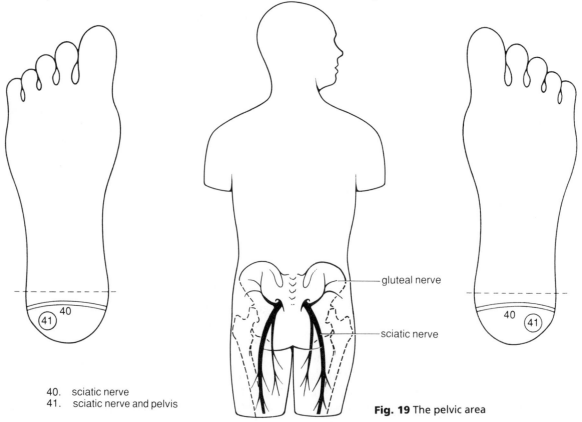

gluteal nerve

sciatic nerve

40. sciatic nerve
41. sciatic nerve and pelvis

Fig. 19 The pelvic area

traverse the pelvic section of the heel. As a result, many congestions here can be traced to meridians and their organs.

The Sciatic Nerves

These are the largest nerves in the body. They arise from the sacral plexus of nerves formed by the lower lumbar and upper sacral spinal nerves. They run from the buttocks down the backs of the thighs to divide just above the knees into two main branches which supply the lower legs: These are actual nerves in the feet as well as reflexes.

The sciatic nerves and reflexes are found on the soles of both feet, in a band about a third of the way down the pad of the heel extending right across the foot.

The outer ankle contains the ovaries/testes reflexes, and the inner ankle contains reflexes of the uterus, prostate, vagina and penis. The reflex points for the Fallopian tubes, lymph drainage area in the groin, vas deferens and seminal vesicles are found in a narrow band running below the outer ankle bone across the top of the foot to the inner ankle bone. The kidney/bladder meridian is situated on both sides up the back of the Achilles tendon.

The Ovaries

These are the female gonads or sex glands. They are small almond-shaped glands about 2 to 3 centimetres long. There are two ovaries – one on

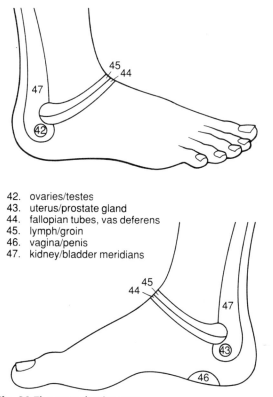

42. ovaries/testes
43. uterus/prostate gland
44. fallopian tubes, vas deferens
45. lymph/groin
46. vagina/penis
47. kidney/bladder meridians

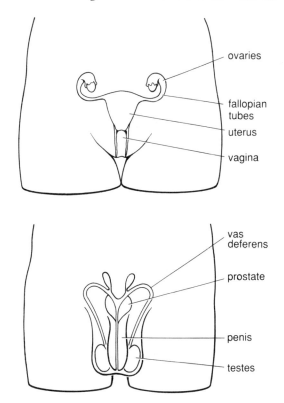

Fig. 20 The reproductive area

each side of the uterus. These are part of the female reproductive system and produce ova as well as the hormones oestrogen and progesterone.

The reflexes are found on both feet on the outer side, midway between the ankle bone and the back of the heel – the right ovary on the right foot, the left ovary on the left foot. The 'helper' area is the heel due to the presence of the meridians.

The Testes

The testes are the male reproductive glands which produce spermatozoa and the male hormone testosterone. There are two testes suspended outside the body in the scrotum – a sac of thin dark-coloured skin which lies behind the penis.

The reflexes are found on males in the same area as the ovaries in females – midway between the outer ankle bone and the heel. The 'helper' area is the heel.

The Uterus

The uterus is a hollow pear-shaped organ about 10 centimetres long, situated in the centre of the pelvic cavity in females. Its function is the nourishment and protection of the foetus during pregnancy and its expulsion at term.

The reflex points are located on both feet on the inside of the ankles, midway on a diagonal line between the ankle bone and the back of the heel. The 'helper' area is the heel.

The Prostate Gland

This gland lies at the base of the bladder in males and surrounds the urethra. It produces thin lubricating fluid which forms part of the semen to aid the transport of sperm cells.

Reflexes are found on both feet in the same place as the uterus reflex on females – midway in a diagonal line between the inner ankle bone and the heel. Again, the heel is the 'helper' area.

The Fallopian Tubes

In females these two tubes, about 10 to 14 centimetres in length, connect the ovaries with the cavity of the uterus. Their function is to conduct the ova expelled from the ovaries during ovulation down to the uterus.

The reflexes are found on both feet. They run across the top of the foot linking the reflex of the uterus to the reflex of the ovaries. This area is usually massaged in conjunction with the reflexes of the ovaries and uterus.

The Seminal Vesicles/Vas Deferens

The seminal vesicles lie next to the prostate and store semen. The vas deferens are a pair of excretory ducts which convey semen from the prostate to the urethra.

The reflexes are located in the same area as the Fallopian tubes in females – across the top of the foot from one ankle bone to the other, linking the prostate and testes reflexes.

THE SPINE – THE INNER FOOT

The inside of each foot is naturally curved to correspond to the spine.

The spine, also known as the backbone or vertebral column, is the central support of the body. It carries the weight of the body and is an important axis of movement. The spine is made up of thirty-three vertebrae. The structure of the bones is arranged in such a way as to give the spine four curves. The spine is divided into five sections from top to bottom: seven cervical vertebrae (including the axis and atlas) = the neck; twelve thoracic vertebrae = the back; five lumbar vertebrae = the loin; five sacral vertebrae = the pelvis; four coccygeal vertebrae = the tail. The vertebrae of the sacrum and coccyx are fused to form two immobile bones. Vertebrae are joined by discs of cartilage and are held in place by ligaments.

The spinal column encloses the spinal cord,

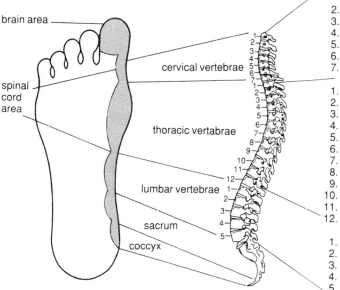

1.	scalp, face, blood supply, head, brain, ears, sympathetic nervous system
2.	sinus, eyes, forehead, tongue, optical nerve
3.	cheeks, teeth, exterior ear, bones in the face
4.	mouth, lips, nose, Eustachian tube
5.	vocal cords, pharynx, glands in the throat
6.	neck muscles, tonsils, shoulders
7.	shoulder, elbow, thyroid gland

1.	forearm, hand, windpipe, gullet
2.	heart valves, heart arteries
3.	chest, lungs, breasts, bronchial pipe
4.	gall bladder and its channels
5.	liver, blood, solar plexus
6.	stomach
7.	duodenum, pancreas
8.	spleen, diaphragm
9.	adrenal glands
10.	kidneys
11.	kidneys, urinary channel
12.	small intestine, circulation, ovaries

1.	large intestine
2.	abdomen, appendix, thigh, ileo-caecal valve
3.	sexual organs, bladder, knee
4.	sciatic nerve, muscles in lower back, prostate
5.	leg, ankle, foot
	sacrum – hip, buttocks
	coccyx – rectum, anus

Fig. 21 The spine

the central channel of the nervous system, which is a continuation of the brain stem. It carries the nerves from the brain to all parts of the body. Associated with each vertebra is a pair of spinal nerves. These nerves arise from the spinal cord and affect the level of the body at which they arise – thoracic nerves affect the thorax, lumbar nerves the lower abdomen and legs. These nerves supply specific organs so any constriction or damage to them will directly affect the connected body parts. The nerve connections of these vertebrae to the tissue, glands and organs are illustrated above.

The spine reflex runs along the inner sides of both feet – half the spine being represented on each foot. The cervical vertebrae reflex runs from the base of the big toenail to the base of the toe (between the first and second joints of the big toe). The thoracic reflex runs along the ball of the foot below the big toe (shoulder to waistline), the arch from the waistline to pelvic line corresponds to the lumbar region, and the

heel line to the base of the heel to the sacrum/coccyx.

THE OUTER FOOT – THE OUTER BODY

The outer edge of the foot corresponds to the outer part of the body – the joints, ligaments

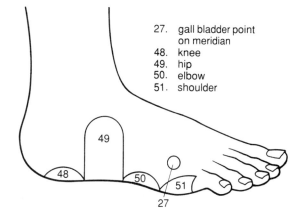

27.	gall bladder point on meridian
48.	knee
49.	hip
50.	elbow
51.	shoulder

Fig. 22 The outer body

and surrounding muscles. From the base of the toe to the diaphragm line = shoulder and upper arm; diaphragm line to waistline = elbow, forearm, wrist and hand; waistline to end of heel = leg, knee and hip.

The Knee

The knee joint joins the upper and lower leg and facilitates movement of the lower limb.

Reflexes are found on both feet on the outer side, just below the bony projection of the ankle bone, which is usually quite prominent on the side of the foot. Again, remember the six meridians run through the knee, so by pinpointing the exact location of the knee pain, one can relate it to a specific meridian and locate the problematic organ.

The Hip

The hip joint is where the thigh bone (femur) meets the pelvis.

The reflex is found on both feet extending towards the toe in front of the knee reflex. It covers an oblong shape, moving out from the line up the side of the foot, in line with the fourth toe. A number of hip problems may be gall bladder related, as the gall bladder meridian passes directly through the hip.

The Elbow and Shoulder

The elbow is the joint between the upper arm and the forearm. It is formed by the humerus above and the radius and ulna below. The shoulder joint is where the bone of the upper arm (humerus) meets the shoulder blade (scapula).

The reflexes to the elbow are situated on both feet on the outer side along the arch and the ball. The shoulder and the surrounding muscles are found on both feet at the base of the fifth toe covering the sole, outer side and top.

TOP OF THE FOOT

Reflexes found on the top of the foot include the

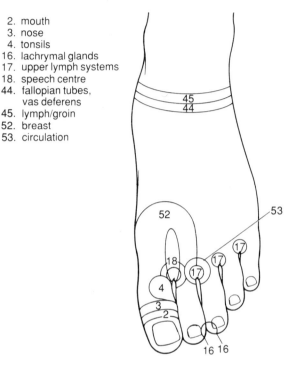

2. mouth
3. nose
4. tonsils
16. lachrymal glands
17. upper lymph systems
18. speech centre
44. fallopian tubes, vas deferens
45. lymph/groin
52. breast
53. circulation

Fig. 23 Circulation and breast

circulation and breasts. Most of the reflexes represented on the soles are also found on the tops of the feet in the meridians.

Breasts

Here it is important to look at the meridians. If there are breast problems, note exactly where these are situated so as to identify the meridian that runs through the affected section of the breast and thereby the problem organ.

Special Circulation Points

These points are to stimulate the heart, circulation and body temperature. They are situated on the top and soles of both feet at the web between the second and third toes. As these are points on the stomach meridian, they have an effect on the thyroid which in turn affects body temperature, heart and circulation.

CHAPTER TWO

Reading the Feet

But is it not sweet with nimble feet
To dance upon the air.
OSCAR WILDE

It is estimated that approximately 80 per cent of adults will develop mostly self-induced foot disorders, even though most people are born with healthy feet. There is a tendency to blame foot problems and deformities – corns, calluses, bunions and the like – on ill-fitting shoes. This is part of the problem – but only part.

Problem areas on the feet relate to problem areas in the body. Which is the cause and which the effect is questionable; it is a 'chicken or egg' situation. Congestions along a meridian or on a reflex – caused by either internal or external factors – will disrupt the body's equilibrium. If the problem is internal, the reflex area and the relevant meridian will be particularly sensitive to excess pressure and friction and more susceptible to the formation of corns, calluses and other problems. However, these external problems cause congestions along the meridians in the same way as internal problems. If these are not dealt with they can have an adverse effect on body parts along the entire meridian, creating imbalance throughout the body.

With the combination of reflexes and meridians, we can look at these problems in a different light and unravel the tales they have to tell about the state of the body as a whole. The areas where problems manifest are particularly significant when integrating the concept of meridians.

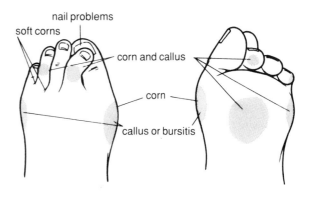

Fig. 24 Foot problems – corns and calluses

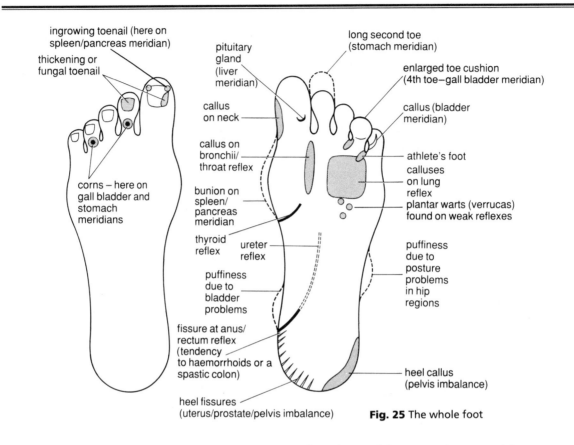

ingrowing toenail (here on spleen/pancreas meridian)

thickening or fungal toenail

corns – here on gall bladder and stomach meridians

pituitary gland (liver meridian)

callus on neck

callus on bronchii/ throat reflex

bunion on spleen/ pancreas meridian

thyroid reflex   ureter reflex

puffiness due to bladder problems

fissure at anus/ rectum reflex (tendency to haemorrhoids or a spastic colon)

heel fissures (uterus/prostate/pelvis imbalance)

long second toe (stomach meridian)

enlarged toe cushion (4th toe–gall bladder meridian)

callus (bladder meridian)

athlete's foot
calluses on lung reflex
plantar warts (verrucas) found on weak reflexes

puffiness due to posture problems in hip regions

heel callus (pelvis imbalance)

Fig. 25 The whole foot

BUNIONS (*HALLUX VALGUS*)

A bunion is a prominence on the head of the metatarsal bone at its junction with the big toe. It is caused by inflammation and swelling of the bursa (bursitis) at that joint. The bursa is a pocket of fluid enclosed in fibrous tissue which surrounds the joints and serves to protect them from friction. In this condition the metatarsal joint becomes enlarged and is therefore subject to pressure and friction from shoes, which further aggravates the problem and damages the skin. Shoes are a major problem in this condition, especially pointed, high-heeled shoes which thrust the foot forward and exert an enormous amount of pressure on the big toe.

As the bunion develops, the big toe moves sideways, constricting and displacing the other toes – particularly the second toe, which is forced out of alignment into a position on top of the big toe. This is known as a hammertoe.

The constriction of the toes can also affect the little toe, forcing it towards the middle of the foot and causing a 'bunionette' on the outer side at the base of the little toe. Bunions look and feel unnatural and usually require surgical removal. Barefooted people are less apt to develop bunions.

HAMMERTOE

This condition often accompanies bunions. It occurs when the medial joints bend so that the toe rises above the other toes and the top joint is almost curled under. Tendons and ligaments contract to such an extent that they pull the front of the toe backward. This affliction is most common on the second toe.

High-arched feet are more inclined to develop hammertoes because of the positioning of the ligaments. Shoes aggravate this condition. Constriction of the foot into narrow shoes can cause foot muscles to waste away by depriving them of movement. Exercises to lengthen the foot tendons and stretch the Achilles tendon will help fight off hammertoes. With age, hammertoes may become more rigid and require surgery to correct.

RIGID TOE (*HALLUX RIGIDUS*)

A rigid toe can be the result of osteoarthritis, injury, obesity or flat feet. The big toe fuses with the metatarsal bone and creates unnatural stiffness. Walking becomes a problem because the big toe has lost its flexibility. As the range of motion decreases, damage mounts. Joint replacement may be the only answer.

Meridians, bunions, hammertoes and rigid toes

Two important meridians are found on the big toe – the spleen/pancreas meridian on the outer side, and the liver meridian on the inner side towards the second toe. Bunions are situated on the pancreas meridian and the thyroid reflex. The internal branch of the spleen/pancreas meridian runs through the thyroid, further indicating their close relationship. Most people with bunions also have problems along the spleen/pancreas meridian or pancreatic disorders, such as problems related to sugar metabolism like a sweet tooth; cravings for stimulants like tea, coffee, cigarettes and alchohol, and constant hunger. They may suffer from depression due to the fact that the thyroid is affected. Many people who have had bunions removed or repaired at an early age often develop thyroid problems in later life. Or vice versa – people with thyroid problems often develop bunions. This is because the underlying causes of the symptom – pancreas and thyroid imbalance – have not been corrected.

Once a bunion has developed in an adult foot it cannot be realigned or straightened without surgery. No exercise or manipulation will push it back. By understanding the connection with the meridians, we can understand the cause of the problem – a pancreas imbalance – and set about rectifying that. This problem is most effectively rectified by a change of diet. Pain caused by bunions can be significantly alleviated with reflexology treatments and a change of diet.

In the condition of a hammertoe, relate where it appears to a meridian. It often occurs on the second toe (stomach meridian) or the fourth toe (gall bladder meridian), and other symptoms may be related to imbalance along these meridians. The rigid toe manifests on the big toe, and therefore relates to the spleen/pancreas and liver meridians.

CALLUSES

Repeated pressure and friction on the skin will cause it to thicken into a callus as a means of protection. Foot calluses are quite common as the skin on the feet is subject to a great deal of pressure, especially from ill-fitting shoes. Calluses grow on flat surfaces and have no nucleus. They most often appear on the weight-bearing part of the foot like the heel or the ball, as well as on the tops of the toes. Calluses also often form on the cushions of the toes – usually the fourth and fifth toes. These particular calluses have the appearance of a thick, sharp 'knife-edge'. The big toe, too, is prone to callus formation. Sports, shoes and long periods of standing may contribute to their development. When a callus appears it is usually a sign of uneven weight distribution.

If this thickening is aggravated by consistent pressure, the build-up of skin will lead to pain and discomfort. Burning sensations in the callus or congestion and swelling under it indicate that it is irritating nerve endings. If severe, it may require surgery, and is easily removed by a chiropodist. If the reason for it forming is not dealt with, it will inevitably recur.

CORNS

Corns, a common foot complaint, also develop as a means of protection. They are one of the most prevalent disorders of the musculoskeletal system. Corns are cone-shaped, have no root, and usually develop on the joints of toes, due to their relative prominence. Toes are particularly sensitive to pressure from shoes.

At the focal point of pressure, the skin hardens and thickens. A corn – basically, a concentrated area of hard skin – forms in the middle of the thickening where the pressure is greatest. Recurrent friction irritates the area, stimulating increased blood supply, which in turn accelerates cell growth. Corns also develop on the soles of the feet in areas of excessive pressure.

Stabbing pain is often characteristic of corns. This occurs when the central 'eye' descends into the tissue and the hard skin exerts secondary pressure on to the sensitive tissue and nerve endings beneath.

Meridians, Corns and Calluses

Corns and calluses may develop on the heel and ball of the foot, and the tops of the toes. It is important to note exactly where these appear and establish on which meridian and reflex they manifest to establish which organs are out of balance. For example, the stomach meridian runs along the second and third toes, and problems here indicate congestions along the stomach meridian. Symptoms like acidity, gastritis, ulcers, appendix and tonsil trouble, sinus, skin problems and breast problems are often found in people with problems on the second and third toes.

The second toe is also often longer than the first toe. This can indicate a genetic weakness in the stomach, which is often inherited but can also be due to deficiencies in the mother's diet during pregnancy. This can cause nutritional deficiencies in the developing embryo, which can later manifest as stomach weakness. If the weakness is genetic, care should always be taken with diet; for example, avoiding excessively acid foods.

Some people have a long callus under the second toe. This relates to the bronchi/throat reflex area. If there is a deep groove in the skin it could also relate to a weakness in the throat, and the person may have a tendency to suffer from throat, tonsil and bronchial problems. The stomach meridian traverses through the throat area – tonsils, thyroid and the throat itself. The stomach meridian is on top of the second toe while the throat and bronchi reflexes are on the soles between the first and second toes. Moving down, the meridian runs underneath the bone region – the thyroid. Many people have a groove or hard callus around the bone which can again be related to an imbalance in the thyroid region; often due to an imbalance in the spleen/pancreas and stomach meridians, as these are closely related. Hard skin over the lung reflex is also a common problem. This can indicate a weak chest. The stomach meridian also runs through the lung area and the gall bladder meridian enters the lung area from the side.

As you can see, it is important to take careful note of where corns and calluses form and refer them to the meridians in order to understand the root cause of the problem.

ATHLETE'S FOOT

Athlete's foot is a fungal infection which usually manifests on the skin between the toes. This is the most common site of infection as the moist, warm conditions stimulate the fungus to multiply. The fungus thrives on keratin – a protein found in the outer layers of the skin. A major symptom of this condition is itching. If this is accompanied by loose, scaly skin surrounding patches of pink, exposed skin, it is a definite sign of infection. Twenty species of fungi may be responsible for athlete's foot, and treatment varies with the type and number of fungi present.

Occasionally a fissure – a split in the skin – may occur at the base of the toes. If this is deep there could be a problem with bleeding. It could also be infected with bacteria and become inflamed if not taken care of. According to medical belief athlete's foot is very easily transmitted to others, particularly where there is communal bathing. Interestingly, men are more predisposed to this affliction than women.

Meridians and Athlete's Foot

Again, it is important to take note of exactly where on the foot the problem is. Athlete's foot will most often manifest between the fourth and fifth toes – the bladder meridian – and can therefore be related to the bladder and its meridian. If between the third and fourth toes, it would be related to the gall bladder meridian.

INGROWING TOENAIL

As anyone who suffers from this problem knows, an ingrowing toenail can be extremely painful and uncomfortable. It is interesting to note that those most often affected by this condition are young people in their teens and twenties. It usually occurs on the big toe when the side of the nail penetrates the skin of the nail groove and becomes embedded in the soft skin tissue. If the wound is hampered in its efforts to heal, it produces granulation tissue which accumulates on the side and top of the nail. This tissue bleeds

very easily and can become infected. Sometimes a callus forms as a protective measure.

Ingrowing toenails can be caused by cutting the nail too short or cutting down the sides of the nail. The correct way to cut a toenail is straight across. Thin, brittle nails and moist skin will increase susceptibility to this problem.

INVOLUTED TOENAIL

An involuted toenail, if not correctly tended, can develop into an ingrowing toenail. This condition occurs when the normal curve of the toenail is so exaggerated that it produces pain down the side of the nail. The exaggerated curve can also encourage the development of corns and calluses on the sides of the nail which will increase discomfort.

It is difficult to cut this type of nail. Cutting down the sides must be avoided, as this will result in the new nail growth forcing its way through the soft skin at the side of the nail, causing an ingrowing toenail.

THICKENED TOENAIL

A toenail will thicken if the nail cell production centre is damaged. This can happen if the nail is persistently rubbed against a shoe over a prolonged period, or if the toenail has sustained injury in an accident. Unfortunately this condition is irreversible. A further complication arises as the nail grows; the new growth curves and is unsightly and uncomfortable. This curvature is known as a 'rams-horn' nail. Many elderly people suffer from this condition.

FUNGAL INFECTION OF THE TOENAIL

This condition – also known as onychomycosis – often accompanies athlete's foot. The fungus penetrates the nail causing it to thicken. If the condition deteriorates, the colour and texture of the nail will also be affected. Warning signs are change of colour of the toenail to a chalky or yellowish shade with a distinct odour. The fungus can spread to affect the entire nail until the nail edge looks granular and acquires a sandlike texture. It is advisable to seek treatment for this condition as soon as possible.

Meridians and Toenail Troubles

With all toenail troubles, it is imperative that meridians are taken into account. Take, for example, ingrowing toenails. This problem is often found in young people and situated on the big toe – the spleen/pancreas meridian. These people usually have a diet high in sugar, junk food, alcohol and cigarettes and many of their problems can be related to sugar metabolism or pancreatic disorders. The big toe is also the head reflex and people with ingrowing toenails often tend to suffer from headaches and migraines.

Check the section on meridians and note which ones run through the area of the foot where the physical deformities and problems are found in order to ascertain which organ is congested and needs correcting.

PLANTAR DIGITAL NEURITIS

Neuritis is the inflammation of a nerve causing pain, tenderness and loss of function. This particular form of neuritis affects the toes, specifically the fourth toe. The pain begins at the web between the third and fourth toes and shoots up into the fourth toe. The sensations experienced in the toe may vary from slight numbness to intense pain, depending on how severely the nerve is affected. This discomfort can be alleviated by massaging the toe. This problem usually occurs in women.

Meridians and Plantar Digital Neuritis

The gall bladder meridian is found on the fourth toe, where this problem is most common. It oc-

curs in many women, and I have witnessed numerous cases where women have this problem around premenstrual time when they often crave chocolates, caffeine and other stimulants which overload the gall bladder. Often, symptoms will indicate other gall bladder related problems.

It can also be associated with hip trouble and can possibly be seen as a puffy area in line with the fourth toe close to the ankle. The gall bladder meridian runs through the hip region, and swelling here may indicate congestions along the gall bladder meridian. In some cases this may manifest as a posture problem which stems from the hip region.

FLAT FEET (*PES PLANUS*)

Flat feet can be caused by numerous factors. They are often inherited but may also develop due to weakness in the joints, 'overloading' the feet or as a result of a long illness. In childhood this condition can occur if growth is too rapid, or if the child is malnourished or overweight. The weaker the foot, the greater the possibility of this condition developing.

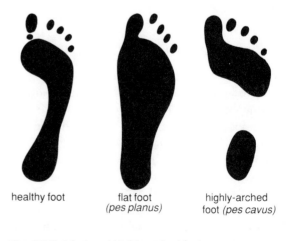

healthy foot   flat foot (pes planus)   highly-arched foot (pes cavus)

Fig. 26 Flat feet and highly arched feet

If not inherited, flat feet can be identified if the ankles lean towards each other. This means that the joint beneath the ankle is out of order, so a weak ankle results. Or the ligaments of the foot may literally collapse because of walking injuries or improper walking habits. The ligaments may lose control and the foot will spread to become square-shaped.

Hallmarks of a fallen arch are fatigue and pain, ranging from a sore arch to aches up to the knee. Apart from causing an unattractive style of walking, flat feet can also affect the spine. The spine becomes more vulnerable as the foot no longer acts as an efficient shock absorber and thus impacts reverberate upward with more force.

Too much standing weakens the ligaments responsible for holding the foot in one piece. As these give way the longitudinal heel-to-toe arch lowers with them; stress registers in the lower back. Back pain is a common sign of this kind of foot trouble. Foot pain or 'burning' soles could indicate strain on the longitudinal arches. Specific exercises may be used to build up muscle strength. Commercial arch supports can provide extra support.

In this condition, overstretching and weakness of both muscles and tendons place a strain on the bone structure. Another problem is that nerves and blood vessels usually protected from contact with the ground by the shape of the arch are now subject to pressure and their condition will deteriorate, affecting the reflexes in this area.

THE HIGHLY ARCHED FOOT
(PES CAVUS)

The highly arched foot is usually stiff which limits manoeuvrability and therefore prevents efficient functioning of the foot. It tends to be transmitted genetically and often only requires well-fitted shoes or metatarsal arch supports to correct the weight-bearing pattern. The head of the metatarsals may ache due to the shape of the foot, and calluses may develop since so much pressure is exerted on that area.

Due to the exaggerated height of the arch, the toes will not have correct contact with the ground when standing. The unnatural shape and position of the toes – they are curled under in a configuration known as a 'clawfoot' – makes them particularly susceptible to external pressures and therefore prone to corns and calluses. Apart from the possibility of hereditary influences, this condition could also be the result of nerve and muscle imbalance. It is often witnessed in the neurological conditions poliomyelitis and spina bifida. These arch problems usually require surgical correction.

The Arch and Reflexology

As a reflexologist I perceive the problem of flat feet as being a rigid spine, indicating that the person is not very supple and could also be inclined to lower back problems. A highly curved arch or curved spine reflex also indicates a spinal problem, and this can affect the upper part of the body in the chest area.

If you press your fist against the lung reflex on the foot and gently push the foot back into the normal position, you will see the spine 'correcting' itself. Any problems relating to the spine reflex indicate that the person may have a tendency to lower back problems, neck tension and congestions in the lung area. As the toes are also often affected, there will be problems related to the meridians found in the toes.

THE HEEL

The heel is subject to immense stress – it bears the brunt of walking and a great deal of body weight. The heel bone is the largest bone in the foot. Walking and running take their toll on this bone, so it has the extra protection of a thick layer of fatty tissue.

HEEL CALLUS

This is formed when areas of skin around the edge of the heel become thicker than usual to protect it from aggravating pressure and friction. It can develop into a painful condition if not dealt with.

HEEL FISSURE

A heel fissure develops when the skin on the edge of the heel splits – usually due to the fact that the skin is excessively dry, and is being pinched in ill-fitting shoes. If the fissure is deep, pain and bleeding can occur. This could also become infected.

HEEL SPUR

This is a bony growth on the underside of the heel bone. Overweight people develop spurs due to excess weight bearing down on the heels. Spurs are the result of a torn longitudinal ligament which bleeds and generates fibrous tissue that ultimately calcifies. It is sometimes accompanied by pain and can become inflamed. Surgery may be necessary.

Meridians, Reflexes and Heel Problems

The heel is the pelvic reflex and problems here will often indicate prostate problems in men and uterus problems in women. Many women have deep cracks in their heel just prior to a hysterectomy and these often heal naturally after the operation. Any other reproductive problems in men and women – infertility, heavy menstrual bleeding and discomfort – can be related to imbalances in the pelvic region. All six main meridians run through this area and organs and meridians can be stimulated by massage here.

Another fissure may occur at the anus/rectum reflex below the inner ankle bone, where the heel meets the arch. This can be related to tendencies to haemorrhoids or a spastic colon.

PLANTAR WARTS

Warts are believed to be caused by a virus. They appear as an elevation of the skin. This protuberance of skin occurs due to an increase in the size of cells of which the skin tissue is composed.

Plantar warts occur on the soles of the feet, and can cause much discomfort.

Meridians, Reflexes and Plantar Warts

Many people suffer from this affliction and find the warts extremely difficult to eradicate – they often reappear after surgical removal. An elderly client had five warts on his heart reflex which had appeared after major heart surgery. Again, observe where they appear and relate the position to a reflex, meridian and organ. Reflexology treatment helps strengthen the problem organ, thus correcting the imbalance. As a result, the warts often disappear.

ECZEMA

This is an acute or chronic inflammatory condition of the skin. It is non-contagious although secondary infection is common. The eruption appears first as papules which become moist and finally form scabs. There is great irritation in the affected part and constitutional disturbances may also be present. If the area affected is dry and scaly it is known as dry eczema. Weeping eczema exhibits a serous exudation from the affected area which precedes drying up.

Meridians, Reflexes and Eczema

The same principle applies here as in the other examples; relate the area where the problem manifests to reflexes, meridians and organs to ascertain the problem area.

ARTHRITIS

There are many types of arthritis – some due to infection, others due to trauma. Since it is a condition affecting the joint line, it favours the large network of bones in the feet. Arthritis causes cartilage to degenerate and the bones to become overgrown or waste away. It can occur in any joint of the body. In most cases it attacks the linings of joints which then become stiff, swollen and painful. Muscles that move joints are unable to work properly, so waste away. Tissues around the joints become inflamed, filled with fluid and painful.

The two common strains of arthritis are osteo-arthritis and rheumatoid arthritis. Osteo-arthritis is a degenerative condition attacking the protective cartilage around bone ends and is aggravated by an impaired blood supply, previous injury or being overweight. It mainly affects the weight-bearing joints and causes much pain. Rheumatoid arthritis is a chronic inflammation, usually of unknown origin. The disease is progressive and incapacitating, owing to the resulting ankylosis (stiffness) and deform-ity of the bones. This condition usually affects the elderly and is more common among women than men. It could be a virus infection, and is often triggered by emotional stress.

GOUT

Gout is a metabolic disease associated with an excess of uric acid in the blood. It is characterized by painful inflammation and swelling of the smaller joints, and generally favours the big toe. Inflammation is accompanied by the deposit of urates around the joints. This condition mostly affects males, and there is a possibility that it is triggered by emotional stress.

Meridians, Reflexes, Arthritis and Gout

As gout favours the big toe, this can be related to the spleen/pancreas and liver meridians, indicating problems with over-acid diet. The other forms of arthritis may manifest anywhere in the foot joints; relate this to reflexes and meridians for further insight into the problem organ. By increasing blood flow to the feet, reflexology can help alleviate the pain and encourage the expulsion of uric acid from the body.

ENLARGED TOES

Sometimes the cushions of the toes become so enlarged they seem deformed. This can occur on any toe but often manifests on the fourth toe – the gall bladder meridian – again indicating imbalances along the meridian or the reflex.

URETER/BLADDER WEAKNESS

The ureter reflex runs across the arch on the sole of the foot, extending from the kidney reflex to the bladder reflex. This can be visible as a clear 'line' in the skin, and indicates a history of kidney/bladder disorders or weakness. The bladder reflex may appear very puffy, again indicating weakness.

CHAPTER THREE

Preparing for a Reflexology Treatment

*. . . They shall lay hands on the sick,
and they shall recover.*

MARK 16:18

A reflexology treatment should be an extremely pleasurable experience. Many people may feel somewhat apprehensive at the prospect of their first reflexology treatment, so it is your responsibility to ensure that the person is made to feel welcome and comfortable. Try to be caring and compassionate and reassure the person that he or she is 'in good hands'. As relaxation is of prime importance in the healing process, the surroundings must be as peaceful and organized as possible. Once the session has begun, all distractions must be avoided. Telephone interruptions or children and dogs rushing in and out will not assist in achieving the desired effect!

People have strange attitudes regarding their feet and many will be embarrassed about the state of their feet. Any insecurities of this type must be dispelled. Feet are a reflexologist's domain – they specialize in feet and are accustomed to seeing them in all shapes, sizes and conditions. The feet represent the body and encompass a wealth of information about one's state of health. They are the key to revealing where imbalances lie and play a vital role in the enhancement of general health and well-being.

MEDICAL HISTORY

At the first treatment, the practitioner begins by taking a thorough medical history. All problems must be noted, not just those troubling the person at the time. This detail is necessary as all problems are relevant in ascertaining a complete health picture.

In order to understand the client and his or her complaint, it is advisable to record a detailed case history. This is useful to refer back to during ensuing treatment to gauge progress. The example of a case history sheet (Fig 27) can serve as a guideline, but obviously you can develop your own to suit your individual requirements.

Guidelines for Compiling a Case History

First note the complaint for which treatment is

Name:_____

Address:_____

_____

Telephone:_____

Complaint: Headaches – forehead, neck tension (bladder), tendency to bladder infections, lower back pain, sinus, feels nauseous when eating rich food (gall bladder), pain around outer breast with menstrual cycle, vaginal infections (candida)

Treatments Tried:

Medication: Painkiller

Blood Pressure: Normal

Bowels: Constipation

Headaches: Forehead/neck

Energy: Feels very tired most of the time

Mind: 'slightly' forgetful

Stress: Has lots of stress at work

Digestion: Heartburn often

Exercise: None
Vitamin Supplements: None
Tongue: Slightly split

Skin/hair/nails: White spots on index finger (colon)

Endocrine: Irregular, heavy and painful menstrual cycle, suffers PMT

Operations: Tonsils, appendix, gall bladder removed

Family History: Mother hepatitis, Father ulcers

Sleep: Erratic

Meridians: Bladder (headaches, eyes, and lower back), stomach (sinus, gall bladder, colon), spleen, pancreas (menstruation, vaginal and breast)

Eyes: Wears glasses

Weight: +-58kg

Diet: Breakfast = cereal and fruits
   Lunch = bread, cheese, tomato
   Supper = meat, vegetables
   Liquids = 6-8 cups of tea during day
   and fruit juice
   Often wine with dinner

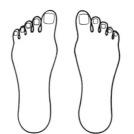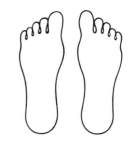

Treatment results:

2nd After 1st treatment, headache was worse for 2 days, felt very tired
3rd Headaches a lot less and less painful, still lower back
4th Menstrual cycle was easier, less pain, only slight PMT, colon fine
5th Bowels moving every day, had no headaches, candida a lot better
6th Headaches still gone, feels more energetic, copes easier with stress
7th Has had no heartburn – feels good.

Fig. 27 A sample case history sheet

being sought. Then take note of all other symptoms and operations in as much detail as possible. If headaches are a symptom, note where these occur – forehead, neck tension and the like – in order to trace them to a specific meridian. If they occur on the bladder meridian, check whether the person has a history of bladder problems. If they occur on the gall bladder meridian, other symptoms may include nausea or intolerance of fatty foods, and thus a gall bladder imbalance may be pin-pointed as the cause.

Check thoroughly through each body system, questioning the functions – digestion, bowels, bladder, and blood pressure. Does the person feel mentally alert? How does he or she cope with stress? Is their energy level depleted? Do they suffer from heartburn or other digestive disorders? What exercise do they take? Observe the skin, hair and nail condition and record this. Check the tongue, as this provides an insight into the condition of the stomach. A clean tongue usually indicates that the digestive system is functioning normally, while a tongue with a white or yellow coating could indicate a congestion or imbalance in the digestive system.

What of the endocrine system? If female, record all problems related to the menstrual cycle – regular, painful, heavy or long menstruation, and pre-menstrual tension symptoms. Also record all previous operations. In this way one can determine which meridians dominate the problems. It is necessary to ask personal questions which may embarrass some clients, but they should be reassured.

It is of vital importance to ask questions in order to fully understand the complaint. Question how the problem developed, how long it has been present, accompanying aches and pains, eating and drinking habits, parents' eating habits, and hereditary tendencies.

It is interesting to observe family history and inherited problems and note how these manifest in related complaints. Often diseases have the same root cause and are situated along the same meridians, but the effects may differ. For example, you may be treating a mother and she decides to bring her child. The mother may suffer breast problems and painful ovaries, while the child suffers from acne and chest weakness – all symptoms which manifest along the stomach meridian. Hereditary dietary indiscretions can often be cited as the main culprit.

It is not wise to force dietary change on a person, but one should try and enlighten them regarding dietary related problems and help steer them towards a more healthy way of eating. Using the stomach meridian as an example, point out problems which can arise from dietary indiscretions. Once they understand the cause of pain and discomfort, they will be more willing to change their ways.

Keep a comprehensive record of each treatment, checking all reactions, both good and bad, as well as changes in general health. The pair of feet in the bottom right-hand corner of the case history example can be useful for recording information. Mark where the problems occur on the feet for easy reference to the meridians.

REFLEXOLOGISTS DON'T...

Reflexologists don't practise medicine. That is the realm of orthodox licensed physicians. Reflexologists *never* diagnose a disease, treat for a specific condition, prescribe or adjust medication. They do not treat specific diseases although reflexology helps eliminate problems caused by specific diseases. By bringing the body back into a state of balance, reflexology treatment can combat a number of disorders. Tender reflexes indicate which parts of the body are congested. This 'diagnosis' is only of parts of the body 'out of balance', not specific named disorders. It is important to be aware of this.

Any attempt to diagnose or prescribe could well land a well-meaning reflexologist in a law court.

THE TREATMENT

Once all the relevant details are noted, the treatment can proceed. As comfort is the first prerequisite, correct positioning of giver and receiver is imperative. The receiver must be seated comfortably, preferably on a soft treatment couch with the head and neck well supported, so that you have eye contact. The lower legs should be well supported with the feet in a comfortable position. Shoes, socks, tights or stockings must be removed and tight garments should be loosened so as not to hinder circulation.

Begin by disinfecting the feet with cotton wool soaked in disinfectant. Alternatively, use a foot spa to which a mild disinfectant is added. Make sure the feet are completely dry prior to commencing treatment. The first physical contact is a gentle stroking movement before you proceed with a general examination of the feet. Every individual is different, as are their feet. Feet reveal a variety of characteristics peculiar to that particular person.

Temperature, static build-up, muscle tone, tissue tone and skin condition, as well as deformities, must all be carefully noted as they provide a more comprehensive picture of the person's problems. Cold, bluish or reddish feet indicate poor circulation. Sweaty feet indicate hormonal imbalance. Dry skin could indicate poor circulation. Swelling and puffiness, especially around the ankles, can be related to a variety of internal problems. Tense feet indicate tension in the body, and limp feet indicate poor muscle tone. Foot deformities are also revealing, and are discussed in detail in the previous chapter on 'Reading the Feet'. Special care must be taken with infectious areas as they could spread to other areas of the foot and to you. These should be covered with a plaster or cotton wool before being carefully worked on. Avoid working on areas where varicose veins are present as this could further damage the veins.

Commence with a full treatment as described in Chapter 4. Working through all the reflexes activates the organs and body systems, and enables you to determine sore reflex points which indicate areas of congestion. Eye contact is important. Most patients will react in some way – usually loudly – when a sore point is located. Some, however, are stubborn and refuse to react. With eye contact, you will be able to ascertain when a sensitive area is located.

The treatment must always be gentle but firm. The receiver should never feel that his or her foot is in a vice-like grip and cannot be withdrawn. This could cause tension from the fear that treatment may be painful. There is a misunderstanding amongst some reflexologists that sensitive reflex points should be worked hard and brutally. This is not advisable, and the patient will probably never return. The pressure should never be more than is comfortable for the person, but sufficiently firm to activate the body's healing potential.

Sensations vary on different parts of the feet depending on the functioning of the related body part. Congested areas will be sensitive – the more sensitive, the more congested. The sensations range from the feeling of something sharp (like a piece of glass) being pressed into the foot, to a dull ache, discomfort, tightness or just firm pressure. Sensitivity varies from person to person. For example, some people may be relatively unhealthy and have insensitive reflexes, while others may be reasonably healthy and have tender reflexes. This also varies from treatment to treatment, depending on factors like stress, mood and time of day. In many cases, a client may feel little or no tenderness at all during the first treatment. This does not necessarily mean that no areas are congested. More often than not, it indicates an energy blockage in the feet which needs to be freed. The feet usually become more sensitive with subsequent treatments.

As treatment progresses, tenderness should diminish, indicating that balance in a problem area has been restored. The treatment should never be painful or cause the person any discomfort; you must adjust pressure to suit them. During treatment, you can return to reflex points already massaged if further stimulation is required. In this way the receiver is not subjected to continuous pressure on one point, which could be painful.

Only in the case of an acute pain should tight, continuous pressure be applied to the area which corresponds to the pain – for example, in cases of headache, sciatica and the like. In these instances apply light pressure for about 15–20 seconds on the corresponding reflex. Increase the pressure until the person is just able to tolerate the pain in the reflex area. In most cases acute pain will disappear within a few minutes.

When executing a full treatment, it is important to complete one body part totally before moving on. Both feet are treated alternately in a smooth, even way, as one foot represents half the body. It is therefore incorrect to massage one foot completely before moving on to the next. No matter what the sensations, treatment is always effective and should leave the person feeling light, tingly and thoroughly pampered.

REACTIONS TO REFLEXOLOGY TREATMENT

People differ, so do reactions – and a recipient must be informed of the possible reactions following treatment. On the whole, reactions immediately after a reflexology treatment are largely pleasant, leaving the client feeling calm and relaxed or energized and rejuvenated. However, there is some bad with the good. Reflexology activates the body's own healing power, so

some form of reaction is inevitable as the body rids itself of toxins. This is referred to as a 'healing crisis' and is a cleansing process. The severity of reactions depends on the degree of imbalance, but should never be too radical. The most common phrase following a first treatment is, 'I have never slept so well!'

Most common reactions are related to the body cleansing itself of toxins, so they manifest in the eliminating systems of the body – the kidneys, bowels, skin and lungs. The following reactions are not unusual:

- Increased urination as the kidneys are stimulated to produce more urine, which may be darker and stronger-smelling due to the toxic content.
- Flatulence and more frequent bowel movements.
- Aggravated skin condition, particularly in conditions which have been suppressed; increased perspiration and pimples.
- Improved skin tone and tissue texture due to improved circulation.
- Increased secretions of the mucous membranes in the nose, mouth and bronchials.
- Disrupted sleep patterns – either deeper or more disturbed sleep.
- Dizziness or nausea.
- A temporary outbreak of a disease which has been suppressed.
- Increased discharge from the vagina in women.
- Feverishness
- Tiredness
- Headaches
- Depression, overwhelming desire to weep.

Whatever the reactions, they are a necessary part of the healing process and will pass. Drinking water – preferably warm, boiled water – in place of other liquids will assist in rapidly flushing the toxins from the system.

LENGTH OF A REFLEXOLOGY TREATMENT

The length of the treatment and number of sessions will vary according to the person and the condition. Their constitution, history and nature of illness, age, body's ability to react to treatment, way of life and attitude have a profound effect on the healing process. Thus, the degree to which the person responds depends as much on her or himself as on the practitioner and treatment.

The first treatment session should take approximately an hour. This is the investigative and exploratory stage which enables you to establish as much as possible about the person. Following treatments would last approximately thirty to fifty minutes, depending on the treatment required. If the session is too short, insufficient stimulus is provided for the body to mobilize its own healing powers; if it is too long, there is a danger of overstimulating which can cause excessive elimination and therefore discomfort.

An effect is often experienced immediately after the first treatment. Generally, results are apparent after three or four treatments – either complete or considerable improvement. Well established disorders will obviously take longer to eradicate than those present for a short time. A course of treatments is recommended for all conditions – even if one session appears to have corrected the problem – to balance the body totally and prevent a recurrence of the disorder. The course should be eight to twelve treatments once or twice a week. For optimum results, two sessions a week are recommended until there is an improvement, then gradually reduce the frequency. A one-off treatment won't correct

problems which have been developing over several years.

If there is no reaction after several sessions, the body could be unreceptive due to external factors such as heavy medication or psychological attitude, blocking therapeutic impulses. As long as reactions are positive, there is value in continuing the treatment.

THE RESPONSIBILITIES OF A REFLEXOLOGIST

The most important asset a proficient reflexologist can have is genuine compassion for the suffering of humanity and a desire to assist in relieving this suffering. But if you intend to become a practising reflexologist, you must approach your task with complete and utter professionalism. A thorough knowledge of the subject – reflexes, meridians, foot structure as well as good basic knowledge of anatomy and physiology – will increase your competence.

A clean, hygienic work space or clinic is necessary to create the correct impression. Grubby, noisy surroundings are hardly the environment in which anyone seeking health care would wish to find themselves. Everything about the reflexologist should give the impression of professionalism – the surroundings, attire and approach. To quote from the *Nei Ching*, a profound work widely referred to as the bible of Chinese Medicine: 'Poor medical workmanship is neglectful and careless and must therefore be combated, because a disease that is not completely cured can easily breed new disease or there can be a relapse of the old disease . . . The most important requirement of the art of healing is that no mistakes or neglect occur.' The *Nei Ching* is discussed in more detail in the section on Chinese Medicine.

Make sure the person fully understands reflexology so they are more comfortable with the procedure. The simplicity of reflexology belies its efficacy, so a thorough knowledge of the subject will give the person confidence in your ability to help him or her. But knowledge alone cannot eliminate disease. Reflexology, as a touch technique centred on the feet, is a relatively intimate practice. The receiver must be made to feel comfortable and 'safe'. They will often feel the need to talk, and should always feel free to do so. Healing, apart from the scientific aspect, is also an art which requires intuitive skills. The art of recognizing the roots of a person's problem and working with him or her to overcome this can only be learnt through experience, practice, self-knowledge and a constant attentiveness to the individual patient.

Try to be an asset to reflexology and present a good example. People will be more impressed and therefore inclined to work with the treatment, if you present a good, healthy image and obviously abide by the health guidelines you suggest. To end on yet another quote from the *Nei Ching*: 'Those who are habitually without disease help to train and to adjust those who are sick, for those who treat should be free from illness. They train the patient to adjust his breathing and in order to train the patient, they act as examples.'

CHAPTER FOUR

The Reflexology Treatment

I have spread my dreams under your feet
Tread softly because you tread on my dreams
WILLIAM BUTLER YEATS

The body is reflected on the feet in a three-dimensional form. Organs overlap each other internally and therefore the same is found on the feet. Many organs are minute and not reflected on the charts, but all are worked on in the step-by-step treatment sequence. In the massage technique I teach, treatment always includes both feet. The reflex areas of both left and right feet are alternately massaged from toes to heel.

Many reflexologists teach the 'thumb walking' technique, and propose working one foot completely before moving on to the next. The main objective of the reflexologist is to stimulate all the reflexes on the feet. As any technique which achieves this result is equally effective, it is up to you to choose which technique works best for you. I have found in my years of practice and teaching that the techniques illustrated here have proved their worth for both practitioner and patient.

The most important aspect of this specific treatment procedure is that both feet are worked through alternately from top to toe. This facilitates a natural flow in the procedure. One foot

represents half a body, and as many organs are paired and found on both sides of the body, it would be wrong to complete one foot at a time. This would mean only half an organ is stimulated. The theory behind alternating feet is to stimulate each organ completely before moving on to the next. In this way, each body part is worked as a unit even though half is on the left foot and half on the right. To execute effective reflexology massage techniques, familiarity with techniques and grips is a necessity. (References to 'right' and 'left' feet mean the receiver's right and left, not the practitioner's.)

HOLDING THE FOOT

The first priority is to learn proper support or the pressure techniques will never be mastered correctly. The hands perform complementary functions throughout the treatment. While one hand presses, the other braces and supports or pushes the foot towards the pressure. The hand applying pressure is referred to as the 'working hand', the other hand, the 'supporting hand'. Neither hand should ever be idle.

The Standard Support Grip

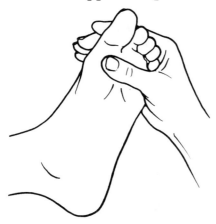

Fig. 28 The Standard Support Grip

There is one main support technique. This is referred to as the *standard support grip*.

Take the foot in the support hand, either from the inside or the outside, the web of the hand between the thumb and the index finger touching the side of the foot, with the four fingers on top of the foot and the thumb on the sole. The support hand must always stay close to the working hand. Whichever grip you use on whatever reflex, always keep the foot bent slightly towards you – never in a tight grip with the toes bent backwards.

PRESSURE TECHNIQUES

The Rotating Thumb Technique

This is the most important technique to master, as it is used to apply pressure to most of the reflexes throughout the treatment procedure. It is combined with finger techniques.

Before working on the feet, try the rotating thumb technique on the palm of your hand. It helps to visualize the object being worked on (hand or foot) divided into small squares, all of

which must be systematically stimulated. As you work, move from square to square, applying pressure and rotation to each square. The movement of the thumb from point to point must be small, moving along progressively, leaving no space between the points covered by the thumb tip.

For this exercise, place the four fingers of the working hand on the back of the hand to be worked on, keeping the thumb free to work on the palm. Bend the thumb from the first joint to between a 75 and 90 degree angle – the angle must ensure that the thumb nail doesn't dig into the flesh. This is the standard position of the 'rotating thumb'. The contact point is the tip of the thumb. Apply firm pressure with the tip of the thumb to the point to be worked on, and rotate the thumb, clockwise or anti-clockwise. Keep the pressure firm and constant and *stay on the square*. Two to three rotations are sufficient. Lift the thumb, move to the next point and repeat the procedure. The basic movement is: press in, rotate, lift, move. The amount of pressure or number of rotations depend on the practitioner and patient.

Observe the movement of the thumb on the working hand. The most visible rotation must be at the second thumb joint – where the meta-

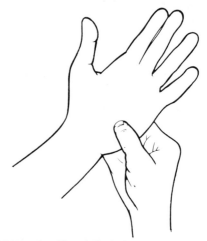

Fig. 29 Rotating Thumb Technique

carpals of the hand join the phalanges of the thumb. Two basic tenets for ease in executing this technique are to keep the thumb bent and the shoulders down. There should be very little strain on the arm muscles, elbows, neck and shoulders.

Furthermore, you will notice how much more pressure can be applied with the thumb in a bent position as opposed to a flat thumb. Ensure that the distance between the thumb and fist is sufficient to allow for easy rotation movements – approximately 2 cm apart. By exercising the correct technique, the treatment procedure should not be at all strenuous for the practitioner. Practise this thumb rotating technique on your hand until you feel completely comfortable with it. Also ensure that you exercise the thumbs on both hands to enable you to work efficiently with either thumb, as it is important to be able to switch hands during the treatment sequence.

Finger Techniques

1. This is used on the sides and tops of the toes. Place the index finger on one side and thumb on the other side of the toe to be worked on. 'Rub' the toe, moving the fingers gently back and forth in opposite directions.

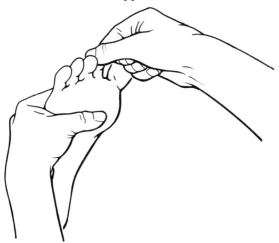

Fig. 30 Finger Technique 1

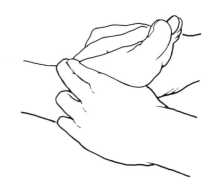

Fig. 31 Finger Technique 2

2. Hands are placed on either side of the foot with the thumbs on the sole and four fingers on top. The index and middle fingers are the working tools, the middle finger usually placed on top of the index finger to create extra leverage. This is used on the Fallopian tubes/vas deferens and lymphatic reflexes which run from the outside ankle bone, along the top of the foot at the ankle joint, to the inside ankle bone. With the fingers, press in, rotate, lift and move as with the 'rotating thumb', moving point by point up both sides until the fingers meet at the centre on top of the foot.

3. Use both hands. Place the hands on either side of the foot, thumbs on the sole forming the support and four fingers on top. The eight fingers are the working tools. Starting from the ankle joint, exert deep, smooth pressure with the fingers massaging down the foot towards the toes, slowly and gently but with firm pressure. Repeat this procedure a few times. Improvize a bit, but massage well. Also use a criss-cross movement with the thumbs on the sole of the foot. This is usually part of the winding down stage of the treatment which culminates in the solar plexus breathing technique. Cream or oil can

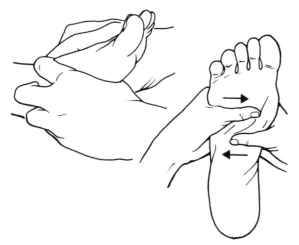

Fig. 32 Finger Technique 3

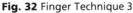

be used at this stage to facilitate easy movement.

Pinch Technique

The support hand cups the foot at the ankle, while the working hand locates the Achilles tendon at the back of the heel and moves up and down the tendon, pinching it gently between the thumb and index finger. (This is used to stimulate the kidney and bladder meridians.)

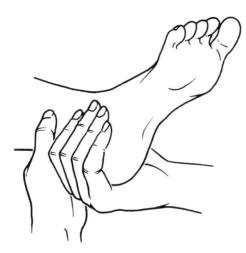

Fig. 33 Pinch Technique

Knead Technique

This is a relatively easy technique, much like kneading bread. It is used mainly on the heel area which is usually rather tough, and therefore needs more pressure for effective stimulation.

Cup the ankle in the palm of the support hand, keeping the heel area free. Make a fist with the working hand, then use the knuckles of the second joint of the fingers to 'knead' the heels as you would dough. This is used for working reflexes in the heel – the sciatic reflex and nerve, and pelvic reflexes.

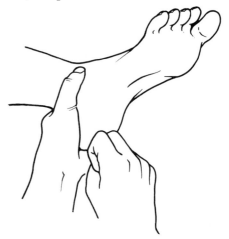

Fig. 34 Knead Technique

These are the main basic finger and thumb techniques used in the treatment procedure. As one of the main benefits of reflexology is the relaxation aspect, it is also important to become familiar with a few basic relaxation techniques.

RELAXATION TECHNIQUES

1 Achilles Tendon Stretch

Cup the heel of one foot so that it rests in the palm of the hand. Grasp the top of the foot near the toes in the standard support grip. Pull the top of the foot towards you, allowing the heel to move backwards, then reverse the procedure, pulling the heel towards you and pushing the

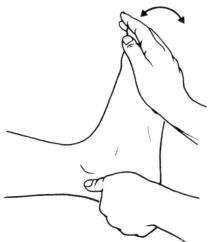

Fig. 35 Achilles Tendon Stretch

top of the foot backwards, so that the bottom of the foot stretches out. Repeat this two or three times on each foot.

2 Ankle Rotation

Cup the back of the ankle of the right foot in the palm of the left (support) hand, with the thumb on the outside of the ankle and the fingers on the inside. Ensure a firm but not tight grasp. Working with the right hand from the inside of the foot, grasp the foot at the base of the big toe in the standard support grip. Hold the foot with equal pressure. Use the hand holding the ankle

joint as a pivot, and rotate the foot with the right hand in 360° circles, first clockwise a few times, then anticlockwise. Work the other foot the same way, alternating hands accordingly.

Do not force the foot into exaggerated circles; manoeuvre it slowly and gently only as far as is comfortable for the receiver. This movement must be carried out smoothly. It affects the entire area of the hip joint and tailbone, relaxes the anus and surrounding area and affects all the lower back muscles.

3 Side to Side

This method of vigorously shaking the foot helps circulation, eases tenderness, and relaxes ankle and calf muscles.

Place your palms on either side of the foot just above the ankles. Keep the hands as relaxed and loose as possible. Do not force the foot to rotate farther than is comfortable for the subject. Roll the foot from side to side by gently moving it back and forth between your hands, which move in opposite directions from each other. Move the hands gradually up the sides of the foot until the entire foot is worked. This is usually executed slowly to release tension, relax the edges of the ankle and calf and stimulate the whole foot.

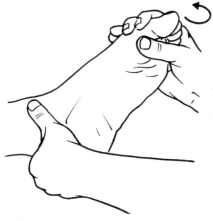

Fig. 36 Ankle Rotation

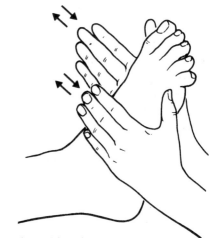

Fig. 37 Side to Side Rub

4 Loosen Ankles

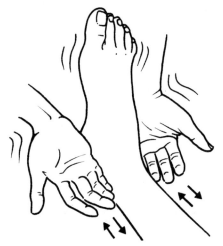

Fig. 38 Loosen the Ankles

Hook the base of both palms above the back sides of the heel so that the palms cover the ankle bones. The ankle joint serves as the pivot point. Move the hands rapidly backwards and forwards in opposite directions to each other, keeping the hands hooked beneath the ankle bones. The foot will shake from side to side when this movement is properly executed.

5 The Spinal Twist

Grasp the foot from the inside of the instep with both hands, fingers on top, thumbs on the sole – the web between the thumb and the index finger on the spinal reflex. The index fingers of each hand should be touching. When working the right foot the right hand starting position will be at the ankle joint on the top of the foot, and vice versa on the left foot. The hand close to the ankle will provide the support. The hand nearest the toes will execute the twisting action. The two hands should be used as a unit, keeping all the fingers together and the hands touching at all times.

Keeping the support hand very steady, twist the working hand up and down. The support hand must remain completely stationary. Then move both hands forward slightly and repeat the twisting action. Continue this movement (grip, twist, reposition, grip, twist, reposition) until you reach the neck reflex area at the base of the big toe. Do not twist both hands at the same time.

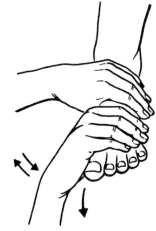

Fig. 39 Spinal Twist

Repeat this on both feet. If the person is tense it may be necessary to repeat a few times. This is a very effective tension reducer enjoyed by most.

6 Wringing the Foot

This is similar to the spinal twist except both hands move in the wringing motion. Grasp the foot in both hands as you would a wet towel and wring gently, each hand twisting in opposite directions. Your elbows should fly up and move when you do this. Move the hands gradually up the foot to 'wring' the entire foot. (See Figure 40.)

7 Rotate All Toes

The principle here is the same as the ankle rotation. It is a relaxation technique which not only increases flexibility of the toes, but releases tension and loosens muscles in the neck and shoulder line.

The big toe is most important here. It

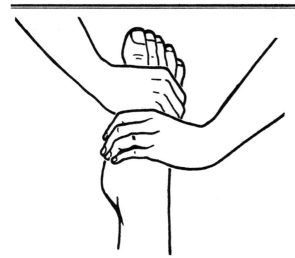

Fig. 40 Wringing the Foot

represents half the head area. The head joins the body as the toe joins the foot, so the area joining the toe to the foot corresponds to the neck.

To execute this procedure begin with the big toe and work through all the toes of one foot before moving on to the other foot. Hold the foot with the support hand in the standard support grip, and with thumb and fingers of the support hand firmly hold the base of the toe you are going to rotate. Hold the toe close to the base joint (metatarsal/phalange joint), with the thumb below, index and third finger on top. Now gently 'lift' the toe in its joint with a slight

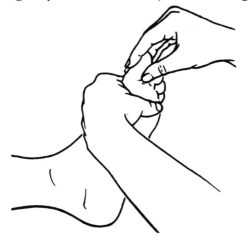

Fig. 41 Rotate all Toes

upward pull, and rotate in 360° circles, clockwise and anticlockwise a few times. Movements must be gentle but firm, the support hand stabilizing each toe individually at the base as it is worked on.

8 Solar Plexus

The solar plexus is referred to as the 'nerve switchboard' of the body, as it is the main storage area for stress. Applying pressure to this reflex will always bring about a feeling of relaxation.

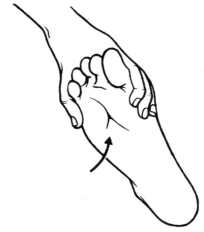

Fig. 42 Finding the solar plexus reflex

To locate the solar plexus reflex, grasp the top of the foot at the metatarsal area and squeeze gently. A depression will appear on the sole of the foot at the centre of the diaphragm line – the midpoint of the base of the ball of the foot. This is the solar plexus reflex.

This technique is applied to both feet simultaneously. Pressure applied to this reflex is usually used as a relaxation technique to complete the treatment but can be used at any time during treatment if necessary.

Take the left foot in the right hand and the right foot in the left hand, fingers on top, thumbs below – from the outside of the foot. Place the tips of the thumbs on the solar plexus

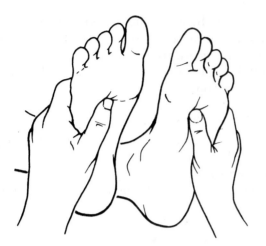

Fig. 43 Solar plexus breathing

reflex. Ask the subject to inhale slowly as you press in on this point and exhale as you release pressure. Do not lose contact with the foot. Repeat this exercise a few times.FIG43.

GRIPS

Grip A

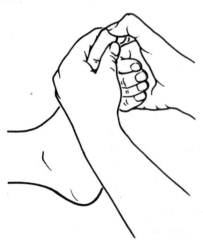

Fig. 44 Grip A – sinus, bronchi, lungs and heart

Make a clenched fist with the working hand, keeping the thumb free. The fist of the working hand will provide additional support on the sole of the foot. The 'rotating thumb' technique is used to exert pressure on the reflex points. The support hand is in the standard support position close to the working hand. With Grip A, the left hand is usually the support hand and the right hand the worker.

Reflexes worked with Grip A

- Sinuses
- Chronic eyes and ears
- Bronchi, lungs and heart

Grip B

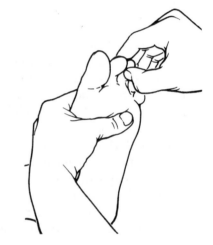

Fig. 45 Grip B – eyes and ears

Here the support hand holds the foot in the standard support grip close to the toes. With the working hand, clasp the foot from above. Place the fingers on the top of the foot pointing towards the ankle. The thumb is then positioned to work under the toes.

Reflexes worked with Grip B

- Pituitary gland
- Brain matter
- Eyes and ears

Grip C

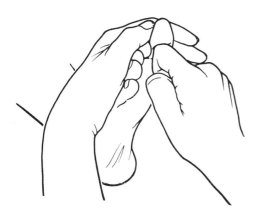

Fig. 46 Grip C – pituitary gland

This is an alternative grip with which to locate and stimulate the pituitary gland if you have trouble with Grip B. Bend the index finger at the second joint and use this as you would the thumb. Find the reflex, press in, rotate clockwise and anti-clockwise a few times, then release pressure when you feel the reflex has been sufficiently stimulated.

Reflexes worked with Grip C
• Pituitary gland

Grip D

Here, the left hand is the support hand and the right hand the working hand on both feet. Cup the arch of the foot in the palm of the support hand. The thumb of the working hand provides extra support on the sole of the foot on the thoracic reflexes, and the index finger is responsible for the rotations on the top of the foot. Place the middle finger on top of the index finger to enable you to exert greater pressure on the lymphatic reflexes.

With the thumb on the sole and fingers on top, reach between the toes till the web between the thumb and index finger touches the web between the big and second toe. Reach as far down the top of the foot as possible with the fingers, and, using the rotation movement as you would with the thumb work point by point towards the webs. When you get to the webs, apply a tight, pinching pressure on the webs as these are important lymphatic reflexes.

Repeat this between each toe, using the grooves between the metatarsal bones as guidelines. Repeat this procedure on both feet.

Reflexes worked with Grip D
• Upper lymphatics

Grip E

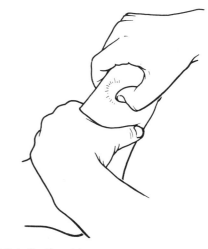

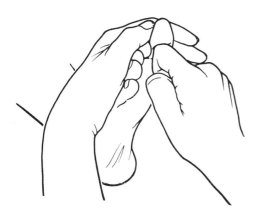

Fig. 47 Grip D – upper lymphatics

Fig. 48 Grip E – thyroid

In this grip, the elbows move out and up into the air to facilitate the angle necessary to get right into the thyroid reflex. This reflex covers the entire area of the ball of the foot at the base of the big toe, but the most important part is found in the half-circle shape at the base of the ball, almost 'under' the bone. To achieve sufficient stimulation, you must get right into the bone at the base of the ball and press 'up and under'.

With the support hand, hold the foot in the standard support grip positioned close to the working hand. The fingers of the working hand grasp the foot from the inside of the instep, fingers on top of the foot from approximately half way down the big toe, and the thumb poised to work the important half-moon section of the thyroid reflex at the base of the ball. With the thumb, press in and up to get right to the bone and use the 'rotating thumb' technique to work around the half-circle of the ball, up to the neck reflex and then cover the section at the base of the big toe.

Reflexes worked with Grip E

- Thyroid
- Parathyroid
- Neck

Grip F

To execute this grip effectively, you must be seated in such a way as to be able to swivel in your seat so as not to be working the foot 'straight on'. When utilizing Grip F always work the outside of the foot with the outer hand and support with the inner hand from the instep; and work the inner side of the foot with the inner hand from the instep and support with the outer hand. The pressure is, as usual, exerted with the 'rotating thumb'.

Imagine each foot divided in half vertically. The object is to work horizontally across both

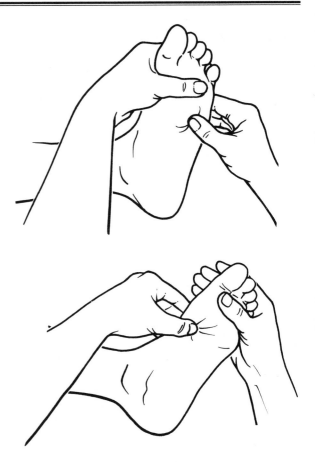

Fig. 49 Grip F – spleen, large intestine and ureter

feet as if they are a single unit, using the imaginary vertical line as the point at which to swap working hands. This may sound slightly confusing at first, but it definitely facilitates a smooth and flowing technique for working the digestive area.

Reflexes worked by Grip F

- Liver/gall bladder
- Stomach, pancreas, duodenum, spleen
- Small intestine, ileo-caecal valve, appendix
- Large intestine
- Kidneys, adrenals, ureters

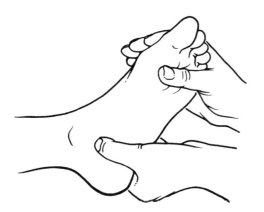

Fig. 50 Grip G – bladder, uterus/prostate, spine and joints

Grip G

For this grip, the foot is cupped in the palm of the working hand, the sole of the foot resting in the palm, leaving the thumb free to execute the 'rotating thumb' technique. The support hand is in the standard support grip. This grip is used mainly for working on the sides of the feet – the spine and bladder on the inner foot, and the knee, hip, elbow and shoulder on the outer foot.

Reflexes worked by Grip G

- Bladder
- Uterus/prostate, ovaries/testes
- Spine
- Knee, hip, elbow, shoulder

Step-by-step Treatment Sequence

The treatment sequence is divided into the same main areas as mentioned in 'Mapping the Feet'.

1 The head and neck area = the toes;
2 the thoracic area = the ball;
3 the abdominal area = the arch;
4 the pelvic area = the heel;
5 the reproductive area = the ankles;
6 the spine = the inner foot;
7 the outer body = the outer foot;
8 circulation = the tops of the feet.

Do not forget – the feet are worked alternately from toe to heel, organ by organ.

Easy Reference Treatment Procedure

Relaxation Techniques
- Achilles tendon stretch
- Ankle rotation
- Loosen ankle
- Side to side
- Wringing the foot
- Rotate all toes

Head and Neck Area – The Toes
- Sinus from big toe to small toe – Grip A
- Pituitary gland – Grip B or C
- Brain matter – Grip B
- Eyes and ears – Grip B
- Sides and tops of toes – Finger Technique 2
- Chronic eyes and ears, and Eustachian tubes – Grip A Upper lymphatics – Grip D

Thoracic Area – The Ball
- Bronchi, lungs and heart – Grip A
- Thyroid – Grip E moving to Grip A
- Neck – Grip A

Abdominal Area – The Arch
- Liver, gall bladder – Grip F
- Stomach, pancreas, duodenum, spleen – Grip F
- Small intestine, ileo-caecal valve, appendix – Grip F
- Large intestine – Grip F
- Kidney, ureter – Grip F
- Bladder – Grip G

Pelvic Area – The Heel
- Pelvis and sciatica – Knead Technique

Reproductive Area – The Ankle
- Prostate/ uterus/ovaries/testes – Grip G
- Fallopian tubes/vas deferens – Finger Technique 1

Spine – Inner Foot
- Spinal twist – Relaxation Technique
- Spine from heel to toe – Grip G

Outer Body – Outer Foot
- Knee, hip, elbow, shoulder – Grip G

Circulation/Lymphatics – Top of Foot
- Lymphatics, breast area, circulation – Finger Technique 3

Relaxation Techniques
- Kidney and bladder meridians – Pinch Technique
- Solar plexus deep breathing – Relaxation Technique

Treatment Sequence Description

This detailed description of the treatment sequence is included to give you a more comprehensive grasp of how to proceed through the full treatment easily and fluidly.

Relaxation

The first step in the treatment procedure is to relax the person, release tension from the ankles and loosen the feet. Begin with the relaxation techniques in the following order:

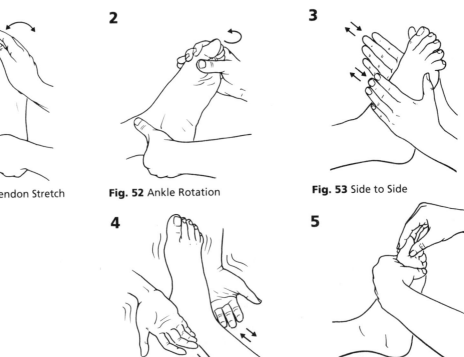

1

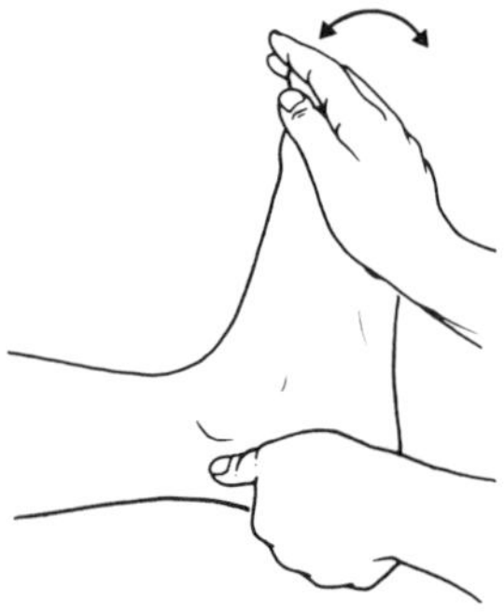

Fig. 51 Achilles Tendon Stretch

2

Fig. 52 Ankle Rotation

3

Fig. 53 Side to Side

4

Fig. 54 Loosen Ankles

5

Fig. 55 Rotate All Toes

Following this, the receiver should feel relaxed, at ease and primed for the full treatment. Remember, whichever grip you use on whatever reflex, always have the foot in a firm but gentle grip, and keep the foot bent slightly towards you.

THE HEAD AND NECK AREA – THE TOES

The toes represent the head and neck area. Reflexes found here include the pituitary gland, pineal gland, hypothalamus, brain matter, eyes and ears, sinuses.

Sinuses

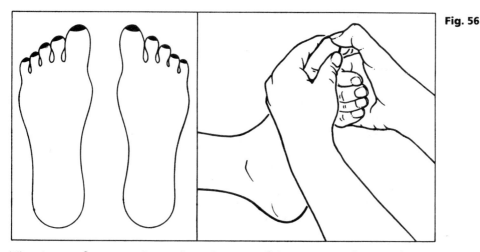

Fig. 56

The sinus reflexes are situated on the tops of the toes. Work these from the big to the small toe, first on one foot, then the other. The technique: the rotating thumb; the grip: Grip A.

Starting on the big toe, apply the 'thumb rotation' technique – press in, rotate, lift and move. The area to cover on each toe would be the equivalent of three to five small 'squares' (mentioned in the practice exercise), depending on the size of the toe. Hold each toe individually with the support hand as you work them to prevent the toes moving and bending.

Pituitary gland, brain matter, eyes and ears

The pituitary gland reflex is situated within the brain reflex on the big toe. The exact point must be located and individually worked on to stimulate the endocrine system. To pinpoint this reflex, look closely at the print of the big toe. The reflex point is situated where the 'whorl' of the print converges into the central point. It often requires a little searching, but is usually found towards the inner side of the toe. Sometimes this reflex is clear as a small mound. A sharp pain marks the site of this reflex, so there will be no mistaking it.

Fig. 57

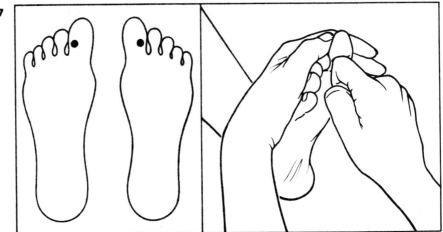

To work this area use Grip B. First pinpoint the pituitary reflex, and with the thumb, press in, rotate and lift. Work this reflex on both feet. Then return to the big toe of the foot worked on first, and work the brain reflex area. Cover the entire area to the base of the big toe using this technique. Then proceed to work on the eye and ear reflexes on the four toes of the same foot, before moving to the next foot to repeat the procedure.

If you have trouble locating and working on the pituitary gland with Grip B, use the alternative, Grip C.

Fig. 58

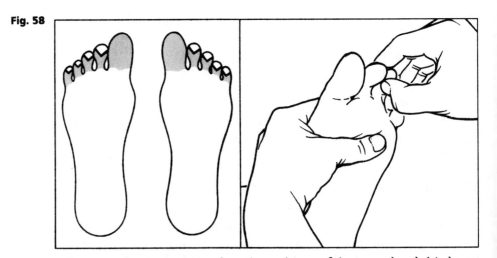

The eye reflexes are situated on the cushions of the second and third toes; the ear reflexes on the cushions of the third and fourth toes. Imagine the cushions of the toes as inverted triangles. The thumb must work on the three points of the triangles on the cushions – two above and one below. Then, without breaking the flow, continue with the rotating thumb down the back of the toe to the base joint (metatarsal/phalange joint). You will often find an undue amount of pain in this area. This may not necessarily relate to imbalances in eyes or ears, but to congestions in the meridians situated in the toes. Always support the toes well as they are worked on to prevent bending.

Sides and Tops of Toes

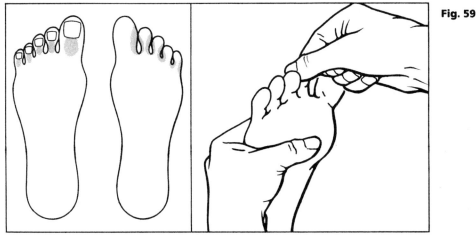

Fig. 59

Imagine the toes as square in shape. Ensure that both sides and top are worked thoroughly. The support hand is in the standard support grip; with the working hand execute Finger Technique 1.

It is important to massage the toes thoroughly, as this will stimulate blood supply to these areas in the toes, as well as to the head and neck reflexes. Most importantly, the six main meridians will be stimulated.

Chronic Eyes and Ears

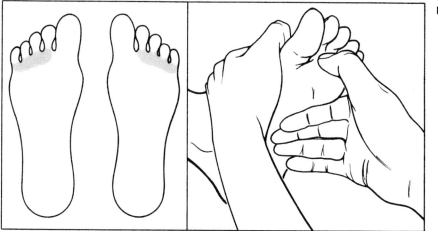

Fig. 60

These reflexes are situated on the sole of the foot along the base of the four toes – eyes, the second and third toes; ears the fourth and fifth toes. This area also includes reflexes to the Eustachian tube.

To work on these reflexes use the standard support grip and Grip A. If you bend the toes fractionally forward with the support hand, a distinct 'shelf' will be visible at the base of the toes. This is the section to be worked on. Grip A is the most effective. The left hand is the support hand for working on both feet – on the right foot, the left hand supports from the outside of the foot and the right hand works from the inside; on the left foot, the left hand supports from the inside of the foot while the right hand works from the outside. With the rotating thumb technique move from point to point along the 'shelf' from the second toe to the fifth toe and then back again. Repeat this procedure on both feet.

Upper lymphatics

Fig. 61

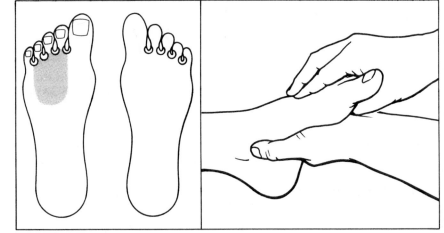

The most important lymphatic reflexes are located in the webs between the toes, but the entire area on the top of the foot – from the ankle joint to the webs – must be worked on for optimum stimulation. To work on these reflexes, use Grip D.

Many people suffer congestions in the lymphatic system, and these reflexes will be sensitive. The reflex between the big and second toes is the throat reflex area and will be particularly sensitive on smokers.

THORACIC AREA – THE BALL

The thoracic area covers the balls of both feet and extends from the base of the toes to the end of the ball. The division between the ball and the arch is clearly demarcated and corresponds to the diaphragm reflex. In the body, the diaphragm separates the thoracic cavity from the abdominal cavity.

Reflexes situated here: lungs, heart, shoulders, oesophagus, bronchi, lymph drainage, thyroid, parathyroid and thymus.

Bronchi, lungs and heart

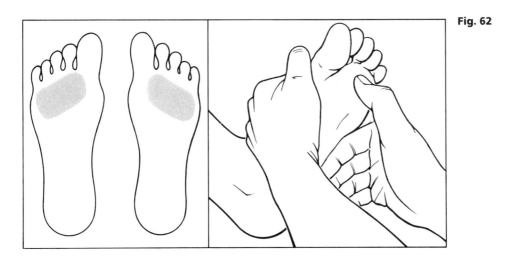

Fig. 62

The bronchi and lung reflexes are situated on the ball in both feet, extending from below the second toe to just beyond the fourth toe. As the heart is a single organ found on the left side of the body, the heart reflex is found on the left foot only.

Using Grip A, start working on the lung area just below the 'shelf' of the chronic eye and ear reflexes. You can move from left to right, right to left, or up and down this area, as long as the entire area is covered. The end of the ball of the foot represents the diaphragm reflex. The heart reflex is lodged in the lung reflex area of the left foot, just above the diaphragm line.

Thyroid, parathyroid and neck

Fig. 63

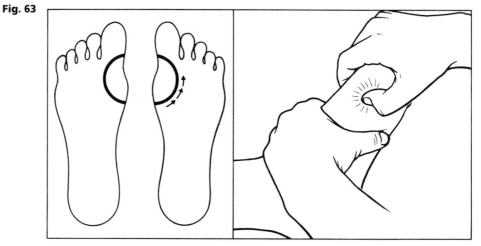

These are situated on both feet, on the ball below the big toe. For this sequence use Grip E. This reflex area is covered in a circular movement – round the base of the ball and up to the base of the big toe, the neck reflex. Cover the entire area thoroughly. The thyroid reflex is often sensitive, so proceed with care.

The Diaphragm

Fig. 64

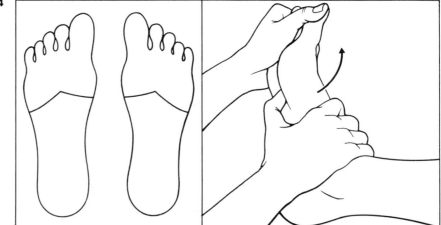

The diaphragm separates the thoracic cavity from the abdominal cavity in the body. Its corresponding reflex separates the ball of the foot from the arch. Use the rotating thumb technique and Grip A to work along this 'line'. The thumb must push up and under the metatarsal bones at a slight angle. With the support hand in the standard support grip, grasp the toes, 'lift' them slightly and pull the foot towards you. This will push the foot on to the thumb. Repeat this procedure on both feet a couple of times to relax the diaphragm.

THE ABDOMINAL AREA – THE ARCH

All the reflexes related to the digestive system are located in the arch of the foot. This section is often very sensitive to pressure. Reflexes here are:

Above the waistline: Right foot – liver, gall bladder, stomach, pancreas, duodenum, kidney, adrenal gland. Left foot – stomach, pancreas, duodenum, spleen, kidney, adrenal gland.

Below the waistline: Right foot – appendix, ileo-caecal valve, ascending colon, transverse colon, small intestine, kidney, ureter, bladder. Left foot – transverse colon, descending colon, sigmoid flexure, rectum, anus, small intestine, kidney, adrenal gland, ureter, bladder.

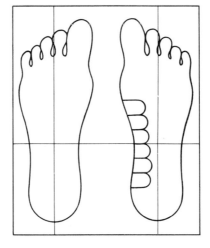

Fig. 65

As this is a rather complex area, with organs close to and overlapping each other, I have devised a method which I find simplifies the locations of the various organ reflexes.

The arch is clearly visible on the sole of the foot – the raised area which extends from the base of the ball to the beginning of the heel. This section of the foot is roughly the equivalent of six thumb widths (of the patient's thumb) measured horizontally. If the practitioner's thumb is approximately the same size as the patient's, the divisions will be perfectly accurate. The first three thumb widths on the inside of the foot cover the reflexes of the stomach, pancreas and duodenum respectively. These end at the waistline. The three measures below the waistline cover the large and small intestine.

Liver and Gall Bladder

Fig. 66

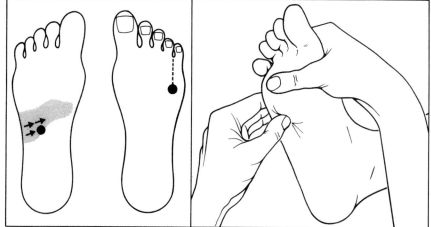

The liver is the largest organ in the body, thus the reflex covers a large area. It is situated on the right foot only. The gall bladder reflex is close to, and often embedded in, the liver reflex – so close as to be almost indistinguishable. To locate the liver reflex imagine a triangle below the lung reflex. One side of the triangle lies at the outer edge of the foot, the other at the diaphragm line. The base cuts diagonally across the arch where the liver reflex merges into those of the stomach, pancreas and duodenum.

The gall bladder reflex is more difficult to locate. Reference to the section on meridians will help clarify this location. Run your finger about 5 centimetres up towards the ankle between the fourth and fifth toes – in the web between the metatarsals. Here you will find a slight indentation which will be sensitive to pressure. This is an acupuncture point on the gall bladder meridian. Once this is located, pinpoint the area directly beneath on the sole of the foot; this is the gall bladder reflex. In some people this is in the middle of the liver reflex.

This exercise is not necessary every time you give a treatment. Use it to differentiate the gall bladder reflex from the liver reflex if there is sensitivity in this area.

Use Grip F to work this area. Support the right foot with the right hand in the standard support grip from the instep of the arch. The left hand is the working hand.

Stomach, Pancreas, Duodenum, Spleen

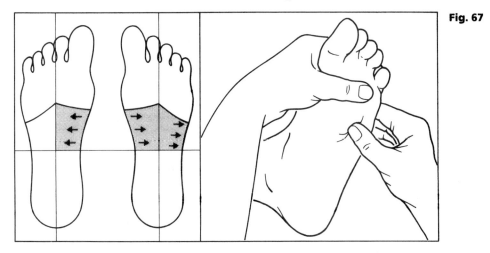

Fig. 67

The stomach, pancreas and duodenum reflexes are found on both feet. The spleen reflex is on the left foot only opposite the liver reflex. To locate the reflexes use the thumb measure rule – the first thumb width pinpoints the stomach reflex; the second, the pancreas reflex, and the third the duodenum reflex, ending on the waistline..

Use Grip F – with the outside hand supporting the outside foot, and the inside hand working the inside of the foot. On the right foot, work inward to the midline. Change hands and work through the stomach, pancreas and duodenum reflexes. Then move to the left foot. Now the right hand is the outside support hand and the left hand works the inside of the foot across the stomach reflex to the halfway mark.

At this point swap hands – support on the inside with the left hand, and work the outside half of the foot with the right hand through the spleen reflex. Repeat the same action to work the pancreas and duodenum reflexes.

Small Intestine, Ileo-Caecal Valve, Appendix, Large Intestine

If you continue with the six thumb measures, the part of the arch which falls under the fourth thumb width is the large intestine reflex. The fifth and sixth thumb widths cover the small intestine reflex. Food is digested

Fig. 68

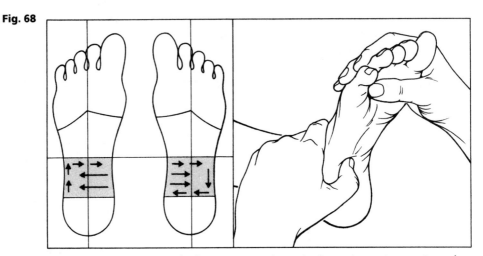

in the small intestine before it moves into the large intestine, so it makes sense to stimulate this area first.

Starting with the right foot, use grip F. Support with the outside hand and work the instep with the inside hand. Work the entire square that falls horizontally in the fifth and sixth thumb width area and vertically to below the fourth toe. There is no need to change hands as the working thumb should be able to stretch far enough across to cover this reflex. With the rotating thumb, move up and down or back and forth, depending on preference. The direction of movement is not vital.

The small intestine joins the large intestine at the ileo-caecal valve below the fourth toe in the sixth thumb width. This valve plays an important part in food digestion. If it is not functioning properly, food particles can enter the large intestine before all the nutrients have been absorbed, or particles from the large intestine may filter back into the small intestine which could cause infection of the appendix. The appendix reflex is slightly below the ileo-caecal valve reflex. A few seconds' pressure can be exerted here with a stationary thumb for extra stimulation.

When work on the small intestine area is completed on the right foot, repeat the procedure on the left foot. Then move back to the right foot to work on the large intestine reflex. This reflex is worked on in the same directions as it functions in the body – up the ascending colon, across the transverse colon and down the descending colon to the rectum. Because food particles can easily become lodged in the corners (flexures), these areas must be worked firmly to stimulate the flow.

Still using Grip F, start on the right foot and the ileo-caecal valve/appendix reflex. The outside left hand works on the outside of the foot, the right hand supports from the instep. Work the rotating thumb up to the liver reflex (hepatic flexure), turn into the transverse colon.

Work with the left hand to the halfway mark, then change to the right hand and support with the left hand.

The transverse colon continues over to the left foot; support with the outside right hand and work with the inside left hand, until you reach the centre of the foot. Then change hands and work with the outside right hand and support with the inside left hand to complete the transverse colon reflex area. Turn below the spleen (splenic flexure) and work down the side of the foot along the descending colon. Curve into the sigmoid flexure and continue to the rectum/anus reflex. Remember to apply extra pressure at the flexures as congestion frequently occurs in these areas. Change working hands whenever necessary for your own comfort.

Once this section is complete, the entire digestive system has been stimulated.

Kidneys, Adrenals, Ureters, Bladder

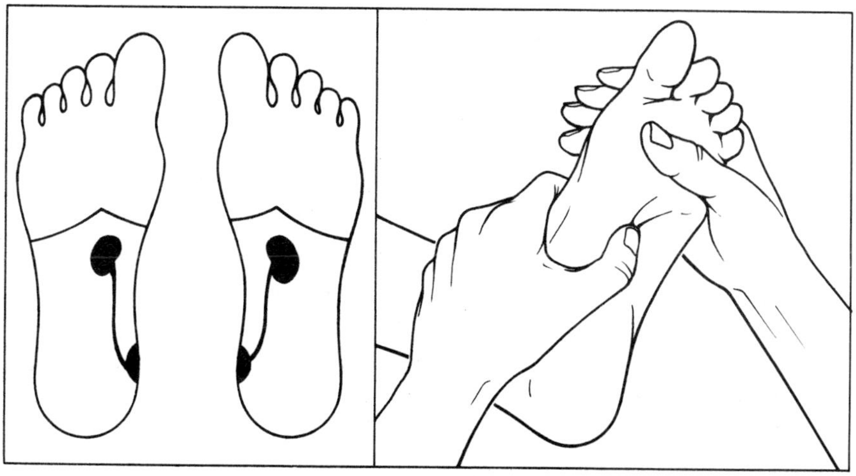

Fig. 69

The kidneys are paired organs, so reflexes are found on both feet. The adrenal gland reflexes are directly above the kidney reflexes so are worked simultaneously with the kidneys.

Again use Grip F. To locate the kidney reflex, first find the solar plexus reflex. This is in the central indentation on the diaphragm line of the ball of the foot. Approximately one thumb measure below this is the kidney reflex. Go in with the thumb, rotate, lift and move down the ureter tube towards the bladder at the edge of the heel.

The ureter reflex is often 'mapped' on the foot, as a curved line descending across the arch towards the bladder reflex under the inner ankle bone. Work this area with Grip F until you reach the bladder reflex, then change to Grip G. The bladder reflex is roughly the size of a

Fig. 70

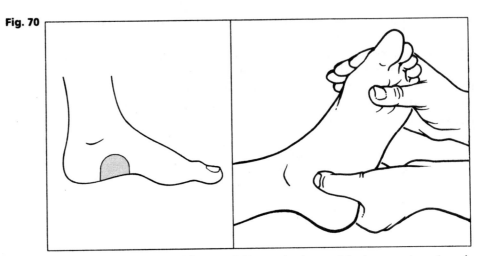

large coin, and should be carefully worked on with the rotating thumb. This area is often puffy, particularly if there is a bladder imbalance.

THE PELVIC AREA – THE HEEL

The pelvic area is the toughest to work on as the skin is often hard, due to the fact that the heel bears the brunt of the body weight when walking. As a result, few people feel any pain in this area. This does not detract from the fact that it is an important area to work well. Many suffer from congestions in the pelvic area and this may be aggravated by the presence of numerous meridians in the heel.

Pelvis and Sciatic Nerve

Fig. 71

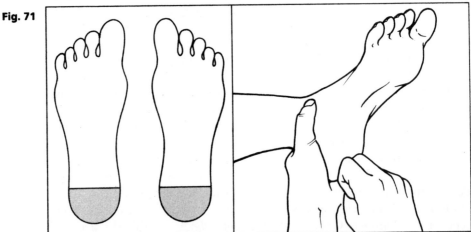

The sciatic reflex and nerve run horizontally across the heel, so will automatically be stimulated as the heel is worked on. The best technique for this area is the Knead Technique. If the client has a very soft heel, knead very gently or use the rotating thumb technique.

REPRODUCTIVE AREA – THE ANKLES

All the reproductive organ reflexes are situated around the ankle area. These are: ovaries, testes, uterus, prostate, Fallopian tubes and vas deferens.

Uterus/Prostate/Ovaries/Testes

Fig. 72

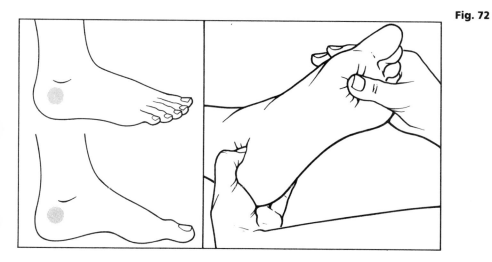

The uterus and prostate reflexes are located on the inner aspect of the foot below the ankle bone. It is important to pinpoint the exact area. To do this, place the tip of the index finger on the ankle bone and the tip of the ring finger on the back corner of the heel. With the middle finger, establish an exact midpoint in a straight line – this is the uterus/prostate reflex.

To work this area, again use Grip G, as with the bladder. The working hand is cupped at the back of the ankle, the support hand holds the foot close to the toes. The area to cover is approximately the size of a large coin. Repeat the procedure on both feet.

The ovaries/testes reflexes are in the same area, but below the outside ankle bone. Locate the reflexes with the same technique described for the uterus/prostate, and use the same working method.

Fallopian Tubes/Vas Deferens

Fig. 73

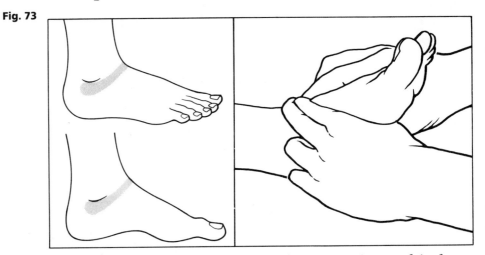

These reflexes run from the inner ankle bone along the top of the foot at the base of the ankle to the outer ankle bone. They are worked with both hands with Finger Technique 2. Alternatively, use Grip G with the working hand doubling as additional support. Work the rotating thumb from the uterus/prostate reflex to the ovaries/testes reflex.

THE SPINE – INNER FOOT

The spine reflex runs the length of the inside of the foot. Treating this reflex will activate blood flow to the spine, loosen vertebrae and muscles in this area, and have a stimulating effect on the entire body by invigorating activity of the nerve impulses.

Begin with the Spinal Twist to loosen the spine.

As the spine represents the midline of the body, the reflex is found in the same area on both feet. The reflex area on each foot corresponds with half the spine. It is imperative to work this area thoroughly and, more often than not, 'tight' areas will be found.

To work the spinal reflex, use Grip G, cupping the foot in the working hand to provide additional support. Start at the tip of the heel and work up the spine to the toes. Use the rotating thumb effectively, loosening each vertebra. If you bend the toes towards you slightly with the support hand, you can see the spine reflex quite clearly. Work along the bony structure on the instep. Do not work directly on the bone, but slightly under it,

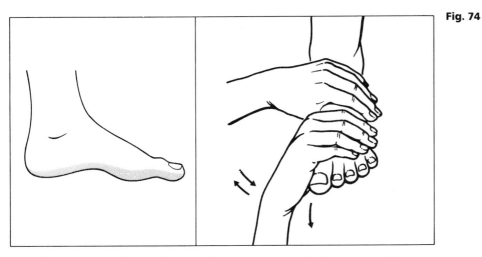

Fig. 74

using it as your guideline. Pay special attention to the base of the big toe as these are the reflexes of the seven cervical vertebrae.

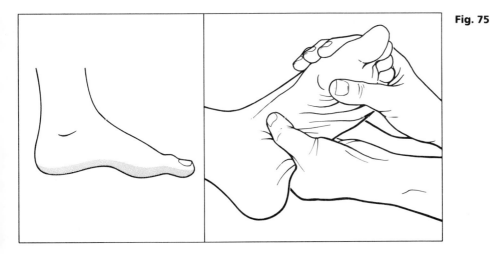

Fig. 75

OUTER BODY – OUTER FOOT

Knee/Hip/Elbow/Shoulder

These reflexes run the length of the outside of the foot. Use Grip G as with the spinal reflex, but with opposite hands. Begin at the tip of the heel and work towards the toes.

The hip reflex is the largest area. It is situated in front of the ovaries/testes reflex near the ankle. Move up the side of the foot until in line with the fourth toe – the gall bladder meridian which runs through

Fig. 76

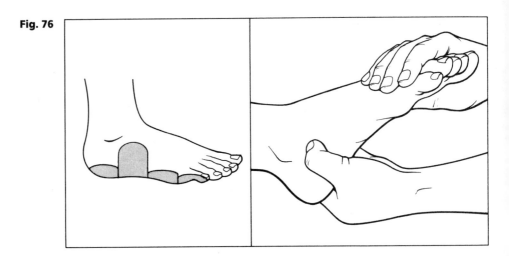

the hip region. This area may be puffy which could indicate hip weakness or posture problems associated with the lower back. Then move back to the edge of the foot and continue working in line to the tip of the little toe. The area at the base of the little toe corresponds to the outside of the shoulder.

CIRCULATION AND BREASTS – TOPS OF THE FEET

Lymphatics

Fig. 77

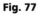

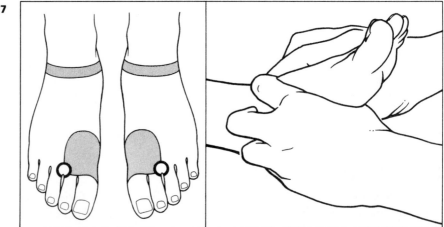

The reflexes for the breasts and circulation are situated on the tops of the feet. As this is part of the winding down stage of the treatment, various relaxing massage techniques can be used. To facilitate smooth and easy movement, some people choose to use herbal cream or oil at this stage. The last three techniques should glide into each other as the final treatment stage.

The best way to work on these reflexes is to use the four fingers simultaneously, as in Finger Technique 3. Repeat the procedure on both feet. This must be a slow, gentle and relaxing movement and move simply and easily into the next movement. Apply extra pressure to the special circulation points in the webs between the second and third toes.

KIDNEY/BLADDER MERIDIANS

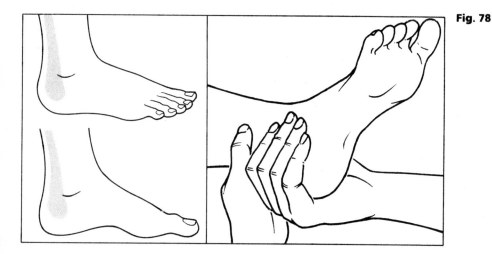

Fig. 78

The kidney meridian runs up the back of the ankle along the Achilles tendon. Stimulating this section is incorporated into the massage begun in the previous movement. Slide the fingers back up the ankles along the Achilles tendon, then apply the Pinch Technique. This area may be extremely sensitive so proceed with care. Pressure here will help clear any congestions in the lower sections of these meridians and thus the related organs.

SOLAR PLEXUS DEEP BREATHING

The solar plexus is referred to as the 'nerve switchboard' of the body and is the main stress storage area. Working on this area will always induce relaxation and can be used at any point during the treatment. The technique to use is described in Relaxation Techniques. It is always used to round off a treatment.

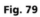 **Fig. 79**

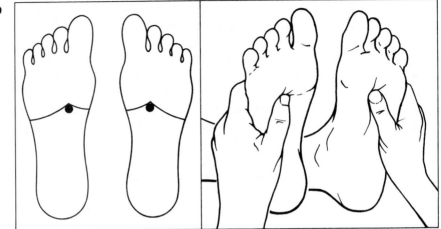

Following treatment, the receiver should sit quietly and relax for a few minutes.

Reflexology Case Histories

The object of reflexology is to stimulate the inherent healing potential of the body. Stimulation of the reflexes and meridians in the feet works to eliminate congestions which may be obstructing the vital energy flow. However, as all the body functions are intricately interrelated it is essential that a complete reflexology treatment is given regardless of the ailment. No part should ever be worked on in isolation, as no problem arises in isolation. For example, a client may seek treatment for shoulder pain, the root cause of which, if you refer to the meridians, is often the small intestine. So, if one concentrates only on the shoulder reflex, the client may experience some relief, but as the root cause of the problem, the small intestine, has been ignored, relief will probably only be transient. When questioning clients, the practitioner usually discovers numerous subsidiary ailments which relate to internal organs, but as they may not be causing any particular discomfort at the time, they may not be mentioned, unless the practitioner prompts the client's memory. Yet they may all be relevant in ascertaining the root of the ailment prevalent at the time. However, even if some important aspect is overlooked, by conducting a full treatment, one stimulates the entire body, activates correct functioning, and

ensures that nothing has been neglected. So, no matter what the complaint, a full reflexology treatment must be given. All the case histories described in this chapter have been successfully treated with reflexology.

BACK PAIN

This is a common affliction in modern society which is greatly alleviated by reflexology treatment. The VacuFlex reflexology system has been found to be particularly effective in treating back pain. A study was conducted in Britain in 1988, and these case histories are recorded in the Appendix on p.185.

OEDEMA

This 65-year-old woman had suffered from chronic water retention in her legs and hips for two years. When she arrived for treatment her legs had swollen to approximately four times their normal size. The skin on her legs was leatherish, dark-brown and pulled tight, with water oozing from the pores. For approximately two months the soles of her feet had been extremely painful, and she had also suffered severe lower back pain, and pain in cervical vertebrae 6 and 7, since 1984. Another painful symptom was temple headaches. Her only treatment was prescribed medication – diuretics, anti-inflammatory drugs and laxatives.

Although her blood pressure was normal, she had very little energy. She felt particularly stressed because she had to urinate so often that it kept her housebound. Previous operations were a by-pass to a leg vein and a cyst removed from her breast. She had suffered two heart attacks three years previously, had a history of thrombosis and could only sleep sitting up.

Following the first treatment, the pain in her legs subsided, the swelling decreased, colouring improved and she was able to decrease her medication from eight tablets a day to one tablet every seven days. After seven treatments her condition had improved so dramatically that her doctor expressed amazement. The patient reported that she had not experienced such a sense of well-being in many years. She is still receiving reflexology treatment for back pain and has experienced significant improvement.

ECZEMA

Eczema was causing this 68-year-old woman extreme distress. It had spread from her hands up her arms past her elbows, and from her feet up her legs past her knees. Patches were raw and bleeding. She also suffered extreme anxiety, tension and arthritis. Medication included anti-depressants, a beta-blocker and sleeping pills. Bowel movements were erratic and blood pressure had dropped considerably in the past two months. Although her mind was alert, her energy level was low. The arthritis was restricted to the joints in her hands and feet. Previous operations – appendectomy and an operation on varicose veins. Her father had a history of chronic kidney problems.

Her elimination following the first two treatments occurred in the form of frequent urination. After the first treatment she experienced extreme exhaustion, but after the second treatment felt very relaxed. The third treatment saw kidney, bladder and bowel movements stabilize, sleeping patterns improve and she generally felt much stronger. By the fourth treatment her eczema had dried up and was receding rapidly. Then an amazing discovery was made. The brown blemishes which she had had on her legs since youth had faded, and by the seventh treatment were barely visible. She adjusted her medication in consultation with her doctor and now reports feeling in total control of her life. She has maintenance treatments periodically.

SINUS

Sinus problems and a spastic colon had plagued this 28-year-old woman since puberty. Other symptoms were two months of lower back pain, a sore throat which had shown no signs of improving after three weeks, and a tendency to colds and flu. Previous operations – tonsillectomy and wisdom teeth extraction.

After one treatment she experienced great relief from the sinus problem. She eliminated for two days in the form of increased urine and bowel movements, and also experienced extreme exhaustion.

A month later she suffered a spastic colon attack. Her doctor prescribed medication but this brought no relief. Twenty hours after the attack she had a reflexology treatment which brought immediate relief. For a period of two months she had treatment fortnightly, then went on to a monthly maintenance programme. The sinus attacks have not recurred at all during this period and her family remarked they have never seen her so cold-free.

KIDNEY STONES

This 49-year-old woman had a medically diagnosed kidney and bladder infection. Tests indicated a lot of blood in the urine, and X-rays revealed one large stone in the ureter and one large plus numerous smaller stones in one kidney. Doctors removed the large stone from the ureter, but left the other stones in the kidneys. The doctor discovered more small stones in the ureter and suggested another treatment. Painkillers were prescribed for the resultant pain but had very little effect.

Her blood pressure was normal; she had a history of constipation and often suffered from headaches on the crown and forehead. Energy level was low, and she suffered from heartburn. Her sleep pattern depended on the amount of pain experienced. Previous operations – hysterectomy and tonsillectomy. This woman also wore glasses.

After the first treatment she experienced acute pain in the lower pelvis. After two treatments X-rays showed no sign of stones in the ureter and no small stones in the kidney. The only stone evident in the X-rays was the large kidney stone. After a total of three reflexology treatments, she no longer needed surgery. To date, no further stones have developed.

MEDICATION SIDE-EFFECTS

This 39-year-old man sought treatment because the medication prescribed by his doctor caused dizziness and nausea. The doctor could find no reason for this and therefore felt he could not treat him. The medication had been prescribed for high cholesterol and fatty tissue lumps – he was informed he would have to continue with this medication for life.

His blood pressure was high, and he was hyperactive. Previous operations – lumpectomies. Although he did not have a history of headaches, he had one on the day of treatment. This deteriorated after treatment. He also experienced tiredness immediately following treatment, but the next day his energy level was back to normal, although a dull headache persisted.

Three treatments later there was no sign of nausea or dizziness. He adjusted his medication of his own accord, and his wife reported that subsequent medical tests revealed his cholesterol levels were normal.

STROKE

While recovering from the anaesthetic following a hysterectomy, this 42-year-old woman had a stroke. She was totally paralysed and 100 per cent blind. Three months later, with the assistance of medical therapy, she recovered 50 per cent of her sight, speech and movement. Her condition remained the same for the following two years.

When reflexology treatment commenced, she had 50 per cent sight, speech and hand movement but very little balance or bladder control. Bowel movements occurred every three to five days. She had tried acupuncture and physiotherapy with no success. Although her blood pressure was normal and her mind active, her movements were very slow. Apart from the hysterectomy mentioned she had not undergone any other operations. Both her parents died of heart attacks.

Drastic results were achieved in this case in a very short period of time. After the first treatment bowel and bladder movements improved. Headaches persisted for a few weeks but gradually subsided by the seventh treatment and did not recur. By the seventh treatment, her sight had improved radically. Her specialist assessed an 80 per cent improvement in sight since her last visit to him. By the fifteenth treatment, her right hand movement had improved to the extent that she could peel potatoes again for the first time since the stroke, and her handwriting improved. During the three months she had received treatment, there had been a steady and definite speech improvement.

'TOTAL WRECK'

For ten years, this 50-year-old man had felt a 'total wreck'. For years he had been in and out of hospital and eventually consulted a psychiatrist. His condition declined steadily. A brain scan revealed nothing.

His condition had started with a closed throat; he couldn't swallow, suffered dizziness and fainting spells. At times he felt a 'pending' heart attack. He saw spots in front of his eyes, couldn't deal with bright light or 'everyday pressure', and suffered from lack of energy. He felt his mind functions were deteriorating. The most severe problem plaguing him was chronic peeling skin – so severe on his hands and feet that he had bleeding, oozing sores. His toenails were thick with fungus. He could not sleep at night as his body would go into spasm. Other symptoms included a history of eye and ear infections, and erratic bowel movement. He was also on heavy medication – strong anti-depressants, sleeping tablets, laxatives, and cortisone creams for his bleeding hands and feet.

Following the first treatment, he experienced extreme exhaustion and eliminated in the form of frequent urination, which was also darker in colour and stronger smelling. Fortnightly treatments proved most effective. After the second treatment there was vast improvement. Although his skin was still flaking, the sores on his hands and feet had dried up. He felt much better and less depressed. At the start of treatment he made the positive contribution of giving up smoking and improving his diet. Each treatment produced marked improvement. After the third treatment he discontinued one of his two anti-depressants. The sores on his hands, the eczema on other areas of his body as well as ear and eye infections cleared up. By the fourth treatment his skin colouring and hair improved, his spirits were high and his outlook on life more positive. He then confessed

that at one stage before he started reflexology treatment, he had been suicidal. He could now play table tennis as his hands were better, and the sores on his feet had healed so well he could again take walks.

After ten fortnightly treatments, he was a different person. His skin no longer flaked and the fungal infection of the toenails had healed. A viral infection of the digestive system caused him a minor setback, but he recovered in as much time as any other healthy person would, and without medication. In his previous state this infection would have landed him back in hospital with complications and additional medication. He had a total of twelve treatments, and is now on a monthly maintenance programme.

FATIGUE

A 27-year-old physician found increasing fatigue made her long hours of work difficult to cope with. Six months prior to seeking reflexology treatment she began to feel lethargic, tired and generally under the weather. An increase of 7lbs in weight, frequent sore throats, spots on the upper chest, forehead, nose and around the mouth, and headaches accompanied the fatigue. Her sight had deteriorated over the past three years and she wore contact lenses occasionally but could not tolerate them for very long as her eyes were very sore. She was sensitive to smoke, suffered sinus problems and flatulence. Sore breasts and candida appeared prior to her period. She found the mornings particularly difficult to handle due to lack of energy, was prone to mood swings, tension and found her concentration poor. Her hands and feet were very cold and purple.

Following the first treatment she was in a bad mood for three days, headachy and tired. Then her concentration improved, she felt more relaxed, lost 2lbs, her throat, colic, flatulence, bowel movement and sinus all improved. She felt much better in the mornings. At the third treatment, her energy was 'brilliant', she had lost another 2lbs, and her moods had improved tremendously. She felt calm and relaxed, and able to cope with her workload.

MENSTRUAL PROBLEMS

Four weeks prior to her first reflexology treatment, this 37-year-old woman had had a miscarriage, apparently due to a low hormone count. This was followed by a D & C two weeks later. She was prone to extreme pre-menstrual tension, painful periods with dark, heavy bleeding and bloating, and during ovulation her ovaries were tender and 'throbbed'. In 1979, pre-cancerous cervical cells were discovered, but these healed. Other symptoms included headaches, sore, swollen eyes which were sensitive to smoke and light, spots around her mouth and cheeks, bad circulation, neck and shoulder pains to the extent that she had trouble leaning forward, her elbows locked and knees were weak, psoriasis on her forehead, sensitive skin, heartburn and colic, bleeding gums, a tendency to cold sores particularly on the bottom lip, constipation and a weak bladder. A year previously she had a ruptured and inflamed trachea. In 1980 doctors had recommended a colon biopsy in an effort to establish if some of her problems stemmed from the colon, but this revealed nothing. She was also prone to severe mood swings, and surges of energy followed by total lethargy. She was not a happy lady!

At the second treatment she was very depressed. Her sinuses were blocked, eyes puffy and she was feeling drained. Her period had started without any prior backache or cramps but she felt bloated. Her urine was dark and she had a bad headache. The spots on her face had improved as well as her neck and shoulders. Her constipation had improved, her gums were not bleeding as much and she had no cold sores.

By the third treatment she was far more cheerful, more alert and energetic. The headaches, elbows, knees, skin, neck, shoulders and heartburn had improved, and her period had been far easier. Over the next two treatments the good results continued.

Two months later she returned feeling very ill and exhausted. She was pregnant. Four treatments during the pregnancy reduced the nausea and boosted her energy levels. A healthy baby was born.

HYPOGLYCAEMIA

In 1988 this 38-year-old man fainted while skiing and was rushed to hospital. He had been diagnosed as having hypoglycaemia eight years previously. Two months later 85 per cent of his pancreas was removed. This didn't solve the problem and tablets were prescribed to decrease insulin production. Other symptoms included swollen feet, puffy eyes, pain in right abdomen, slight constipation, weak bladder, cold sweats at night. Three years previously he had had gout in his big toe and had suffered three attacks since. Since his operation his knees were so painful he could not stand easily, felt tired, unfit, depressed and tense. He also smoked forty cigarettes a week.

He gave up smoking after the first treatment, and the main reaction to treatment was a headache which lasted four days. Although his eyes and feet were still swollen and his knees stiff, his constipation, lower back pain, and night sweats had stopped. He generally felt much happier. By the fourth treatment he felt much better and calmer. He continued with weekly treatments and is now cycling, horse riding, diving and jogging. He is very happy and positive with no aches and pains.

PSORIASIS

This 23-year-old man developed a problem with psoriasis when he was 4 years old. It now covered his chest, stomach, back, behind his ears, forehead, knees, elbows and inner thighs. Two years previously it had been so severe he had gone on a special diet. This helped but he had to give it up as he lost too much weight. He had a poor appetite, was bloated after eating, had stiff, painful neck and shoulder blades especially on waking and his ears felt full and waxy. Weak sensitive eyes were also troublesome, being very painful when moving from light to dark, twitching and losing focus when reading. He also suffered extreme mood fluctuations, and tended to lethargy.

The second treatment saw him very tired, depressed and out of breath, with little improvement in symptoms. But by the third treatment the psoriasis had visibly improved, as well as appetite and energy level. Although his eyes were still sensitive, the headaches were milder, and he felt calmer and happier. At the fifth treatment all the symptoms had improved. He had a four-month break and then fourteen regular treatments by which time his skin was almost perfect, he'd picked up weight, was revitalized and had no aches and pains at all.

INSOMNIA

For ten years prior to seeking reflexology treatment, this 58-year-old man had suffered from very disrupted sleep patterns – waking up every night and reading for a few hours. Although his energy level was good, he was apt to doze off around lunch time and in the evenings. A tennis injury seven years before had resulted in a frozen shoulder for which he was on medication – osteopathic help had not solved the problem. Neck pressure caused terrible headaches over the eye area. Another sporting injury resulted in torn knee ligaments, and therefore stiffness when walking downstairs. He had had a fungal infection in the nails for seven to eight years for which he had taken medication, but the side-effects caused diarrhoea so

he discontinued the medication. His eyesight was deteriorating and he had watering eyes and ringing ears. He was also a terrible worrier, very fussy and had difficulty forming relationships.

At the second treatment he was far more relaxed. The noise in his ears had ceased, sleep had improved, he was dozing off less often, shoulder and neck were fine, no headaches, eyes had stopped watering, knees had improved and he was a lot less worried. By the fifth treatment he was sleeping peacefully right through the night. His knees were fine even during a tennis tournament. He felt completely relaxed and revitalized.

HEADACHES

This 34-year-old woman had suffered from headaches all her life. They would start around the eyes, spread over the head and into the neck. She felt exhausted, her memory was poor and concentration terrible. Other symptoms included occasional ringing in the ears, low back pain, neck tension, dry lips, breathlessness, and for nine months she had mild cystitis. Her left leg was also very uncomfortable and she experienced pain in the left hip.

At the second treatment she was coming down with flu. Her headaches were more severe, tiredness had increased and lower back and hip pain had worsened. However, the ringing in the ears had stopped, her left leg had improved and the neck tension was gone. She felt much 'lighter'. By the fourth treatment she was feeling great. The headaches had stopped, energy level had risen and the other symptoms had improved considerably.

LYMPHOEDEMA

The doctor had diagnosed this 36-year-old woman as having lymphoedema – her left ankle was always very swollen but this had deteriorated over the past six months. Prior to her periods she experienced acute pre-menstrual tension – irritability, aggressiveness, headaches and tender breasts – as well as a craving for sweets. Other symptoms included sore eyes, nose congestion, frequent sneezing, dull buzzing in the ears, a tendency to sore throats, flatulence and bloating, weak bladder, shoulder tension, aching 'tingling' legs and low back. In the mornings she felt very tired and experienced an energy slump at about two o'clock in the afternoon. She was prone to radical mood swings.

Following the first treatment her ankles were less swollen, headaches had improved, she found waking in the morning easier, nasal congestion and eyes had improved, and she had no buzzing in the ears or sore throats. Flatulence, bloating and low back pain had improved as well as her knees and legs. She also lost 5lbs and suffered no mood swings. By the fifth treatment her period started with no pre-menstrual tension at all, and her ankle problems continued to improve.

ME (CHRONIC FATIGUE SYNDROME)

Up to two years prior to his first reflexology treatment, this 39-year-old man had enjoyed good health. He suddenly began to feel very ill, and experience panic attacks and fainting spells. His white blood cell count was very high, and he had not been well since.

Nine months previously he had begun to experience giddiness when tilting his head, for which he was prescribed stabilizing tablets that only aggravated the situation. He felt more peculiar every day but another blood test revealed his white cell count had returned to normal. He had great difficulty getting out of bed, experienced weakness and exhaustion and had been off work for six months. His chest, bladder and stomach were weak and he often suffered from pins and needles in his left hand. Following numerous tests and a brain scan he was diagnosed as having ME.

After the first treatment he felt tired and light-headed, but by the third treatment he felt more optimistic and cheerful and no longer felt the need to sleep during the day. Over the course of treatment his health was up and down, but after twenty treatments he was sufficiently recovered to return to work. Although he still suffered some aches and pains, his concentration, memory and energy level had improved, the main problematic symptoms had been eliminated and he felt he was once again able to cope.

CHAPTER SIX

Foot Care

Healthy Feet can hear the very heart of Mother Earth.

SITTING BULL

In the average seventy-year lifespan, out feet cover some 70,000 miles. This is the equivalent of 2.5 times around the world and averages 1000 miles a year.[1] This is extremely impressive, so considering how much our feet do for us, how much do we do for them in return? Very little. In the Western world, millions of people are treated annually for foot problems and deformities. Despite these distressing statistics, very little attention is afforded to proper foot care.

A health-conscious person may pay a great deal of attention to diet, avoiding the hazards of food additives, smoking and other forms of pollution, but is often completely unaware of the health damage caused by ill-fitting shoes. Most people are born with healthy feet, but statistics indicate that 80 per cent of adults will develop foot disorders at some point – the majority of these being self-induced.

Foot disorders disrupt our centre of gravity and can cause knee, leg and calf pain as well as severe backache and knee instability. As meridians and reflexes are also affected, problems can arise in corresponding body parts. Most foot disorders can be avoided and corrected with proper foot and health care.

REFLEXOLOGY AS PREVENTIVE THERAPY

Health-threatening dangers lurk around every corner in our modern environment: polluted land, air and water, contaminated food, contaminated environment. Add to this the stress of our day-to-day lives – bad diet, attitudes and lifestyle – and we have a potentially lethal cocktail designed to encourage disease. Most people wait until disease rears its ugly head before seeking help but it is infinitely more sensible to listen to the body's warning signals and take action early. Apart from caring for the body by eating more sensibly, exercising and calming the mind and body with relaxation and meditation techniques, occasional visits to a reflexologist as extra 'maintenance' can be of enormous benefit.

Preventive therapy is useful for people who

have completed a course of treatment and want to avoid any problem re-emerging, as well as for those who may not have any acute symptoms but realize the need for preventive action. Treatments at regular intervals can assist the body in maintaining a balanced state, and prevent the possibility of slight imbalances becoming troublesome.

The intervals between treatments will vary from person to person and may involve weeks or months. For best results, treatment should be applied in the correct manner by a trained therapist, but it can also be beneficial to work on certain reflexes oneself between sessions to act as a boost to the treatment. To quote Avi Grinberg from his book *Holistic Reflexology*: 'The truly successful treatment is not the one that saves the person from a condition that is in its advanced stage, but is one that prevents its development into a serious or chronic condition.'

Healing is always a possibility. There are many components in healing beyond the physical. So, with reflexology, even though we may be working on the physical level, we still need to be quite conscious of the mental, emotional and spiritual levels. Healing usually occurs when these three elements are recognized. There needs to be a balance between the body and its environment, the physical, emotional and mental conditions. In this climate, effective, enduring healing can occur.

Rest, a change of environment, or, most importantly, a change in attitude can aid in restoring balance. Often we do not get the rest we would like, or cannot change our environment, but a change in attitude can have remarkable results and is of vital importance to the healing process. Many people feel the need to talk during a treatment session. By talking about what is happening in their lives, they can sometimes come to a new understanding of their problems. Or perhaps the reflexologist can suggest a different perspective or approach to a problem in a non-judgemental way. This helps the person relax and see that a change in attitude is possible. He or she may perceive things differently and make the necessary changes in their environment. This in turn will help the body, mind and spirit to function in a state of balance or homoeostasis.

SELF-TREATMENT WITH REFLEXOLOGY

Self-treatment can be awkward and arduous, but if you are willing to devote the time and energy to yourself, it is certainly worth the effort.

There are disadvantages to self-treatment. First and foremost, all-important relaxation is impossible to achieve. And second, the vital energy exchange between subject and practitioner – which plays a major role in the success of the treatment – is lacking, as you are both practitioner and patient at the same time. Self-treatment is therefore only useful as a means of preventive treatment, general health care and first aid (to achieve quick relief from a condition), until you can arrange for professional assistance. This form of treatment could never be as effective as, or replace, professional treatment from a trained practitioner.

However, for those willing and able to devote the time and energy to themselves, self-treatment can have beneficial results. It can be undertaken by anyone reasonably agile. One should be able to comfortably sit cross-legged or raise one foot on to the opposite knee.

Comfortable seating is the first prerequisite. Sit on a chair or cross-legged on the floor or bed with cushions behind your back. If you are aware which reflexes are out of balance, work specifically on those. Remember, it is difficult to assess your own reflexes accurately. It is obviously best to work slowly and gently through the whole treatment sequence described in

Chapter 4. An alternative is to concentrate treatment on the toes, in which sections of the six main meridians are present. Stimulating these can be extremely beneficial. It is important to be as relaxed as possible, with no tension in the legs.

A full treatment will take approximately an hour, which may be a bit much for many to contemplate. However, treatment of appropriate reflex points can be used to relieve headaches, migraines, muscle aches and other transient conditions. At the end of a treatment always take the time to sit or lie back for approximately fifteen minutes and relax with breathing techniques.

FOOT CARE

It pays to take care of your feet. A bit of time and attention will not only keep your feet looking good, but will have further health benefits. Having now seen that every part of the foot represents a part of the body, the relevance of treating the feet with care and kindness is obvious. Of primary importance is good hygiene. Foot hygiene focuses on washing the feet thoroughly every day to remove dead skin and eliminate bacteria.

The average foot gives off about half a cup of moisture a day. The skin becomes soft and soggy as a result of the moisture, making it easier for friction to cause blisters, for chemicals to leach from shoes and cause contact dermatitis, and for athlete's foot and other forms of fungi to take hold.

The most common problem from all that moisture is bromhidrosis – a scientific term for smelly feet. This occurs because the foot's warmth and sweat provide choice growing conditions for bacteria. Good foot hygiene will help combat this by reducing perspiration. Perspiration can also be reduced by paying special attention to the type of footwear you use.

These are a few basic foot care hints:

- Wash your feet carefully and dry thoroughly, especially between the toes.
- Allow your feet to 'air out'. Don't keep them locked up in shoes all the time.
- Trim your toenails straight across.
- Use creams to keep the skin supple and powders on your feet to absorb extra moisture and prevent infection and odour.
- Regular pedicures are very beneficial.

Regular washing and careful drying will prevent cracks developing. A pumice stone and creams will help soften hardened areas. Problems such as corns, verrucas and athlete's foot should be attended to, and a chiropodist consulted for persistent problems.

Feet should also be kept warm and comfortable at all times. There is a good reason for this. Changes in foot temperature can exacerbate health problems. I am at present living in a warm sub-tropical climate, where I have found sinus, runny noses, chest problems and bladder weakness to be common problems amongst children. Due to the high outdoor temperatures, air-conditioners are common. Thus children are constantly moving between the hot outdoors and cool indoors, usually barefoot. A rapid drop in foot temperature will have an adverse effect on the reflexes and meridians, and thereby the related organs.

A CASE HISTORY

A young male client suffered constant sinus and chest problems, and asthma attacks. He responded well to reflexology treatments, but there was a constant recurrence of asthma attacks and often a slight cold. I checked his daily routine. On rising in the morning he would go straight from the warm bed into the garden (on to the cool, dew-covered grass) to let out the dogs and collect his newspaper. He would then go back indoors for a shower and walk around barefoot on tiled floors. The rapid variations in foot temperature were having an adverse effect on his entire body, causing this propensity to colds and asthma. I recommended that he wear shoes to keep his foot temperature constant and his condition improved tremendously.

SHOES, SOCKS AND STOCKINGS

Most adults have abused feet, caused mainly by ill-fitting shoes. There are no shoes on the market that conform to the outline of the human foot – this is obvious if you just place your shoe beside your foot and compare the shape. Another factor is that no-one has two identical feet – one foot is always slightly larger than the other. High-heeled shoes are probably the worst culprits as they affect the body weight, balance and, thereby, the spine. Synthetic shoes should also be avoided as they do not ventilate, thus increasing the risk of fungal infection. Rubber and plastic shoes will stifle the feet. Low-heeled, lightweight, leather or natural fibre shoes are the best. So choose your shoes carefully; your health depends on it.[2]

Socks and stockings made of synthetic materials should also be avoided, as they increase the likelihood of sweating. Choose cotton and wool rather than nylon.

FEET TREATS

Foot Baths

Famous herbalist and healer Maurice Messegue recommended herbal foot baths as an essential part of his treatment. He believed treatment by osmosis to be most effective as the main healing ingredients rapidly penetrate the skin and sometimes reach the affected areas faster than if the same ingredients are taken internally. He chose foot and hand baths over hip and full baths as they are easy to prepare and because the

hands and feet are the most receptive parts of the body.

Baths can be prepared with dried herbs or aromatherapy oils infused in boiling water. Foot baths should be taken as hot as possible (but not boiling), first thing in the morning on an empty stomach, and should not last for more than eight minutes.

Creams and Oils

A therapist may apply herbal ointment or oil to stimulate circulation and relax the client at the end of a treatment. It is a good idea to pamper your feet like this at regular intervals – either after a self-treatment or merely to relax and revitalize your feet. There are numerous foot creams on the market, but it is preferable to use something natural and herbal like aromatherapy oils or herbal creams as they contain beneficial healing properties.

Chemical foot sprays should be avoided. They clog the pores and stop the feet ridding themselves and the body of excretions from the sweat glands. It is not wise to suppress the ability of the body to perspire through the feet. Excessive sweating is an indication of imbalance and should not be ignored.

Reflexology Shoes

These shoes have 'quills' which massage the foot and stimulate the reflexes and meridians while walking. Using these is not a replacement for reflexology, but is beneficial in that they promote lymphatic drainage and circulation to the feet. They should be used in moderation as exaggerated use can overstimulate reflexes and cause discomfort. They should be taken off as soon as there is any discomfort. It may be advisable to wear the shoes for approximately 20 minutes daily for the first week or two, to build up the resilience of the reflexes in the foot and the corresponding body organs, before progressing to wearing them for longer periods.

Other Foot Aids

There are numerous 'foot aids' available on the market today: reflexology mats similar to the shoes; wood or plastic rollers; brushes and electrically operated gadgets and many types of balls. As with the shoes, these help tone and relax the foot and increase lymphatic drainage and circulation but should be used in moderation to prevent overstimulation. They are effective for health maintenance, but not for treating specific problems.

When using any of the 'roller' type aids, roll them in a uniform way with an even, light pressure over the entire foot – bottom and sides. No special emphasis need be placed on any particular reflexes. Apply this rolling therapy every day for approximately ten minutes per foot.

Exercise

Correct and regular foot exercise will not only keep the feet in good shape, but can also combat deformities. Specific exercises are often pre-scribed by physiotherapists for chronic foot disorders, with excellent results.

There are some simple, easy exercises which can be done at home or the office, which will be beneficial to the feet and should be practised whenever the opportunity arises:

- Rotate the foot to limber it up.
- To tone up ligaments and tendons, pick up marbles with the toes.
- To strengthen the arches, stand with your feet flat on the floor and curl the toes under.

Walking is one of the best and simplest forms of exercise – walk barefoot as often as possible to allow your feet to recover from the confinement of shoes. Barefooted people are less likely to develop foot deformities. A natural foot massage is by far the best – and probably more effective than any gadget. A barefoot walk on the beach, grass or bare earth brings the feet into contact with the earth and the energies that flow through it to provide a revitalizing, energizing and natural massage.

Section four

THE PRINCIPLES OF CHINESE MEDICINE

Tao produced the One.
The One produced the two.
The two produced the three.
And the three produced ten thousand things.
The ten thousand things carry the Yin
   and embrace the Yang
   and through the blending of the Qi
   they achieve harmony.

LAO TZU

To many Westerners, Chinese medicine probably seems as inscrutable as the Orientals themselves because it is based on philosophies and terminology so vastly different from Western medicine. The terminology is so symbolic and poetic that it resembles ancient allegorical storytelling more than medical discourse. This alone makes it relatively imcomprehensible to Western minds. Western medical tradition finds it difficult to understand illness described in terms of 'dampness', 'wind', 'heat', 'cold' and 'dryness', while traditional Chinese medical men are equally bemused by many Western medical concepts. They do not, for example, recognize the Western concept of the nervous system, or Western anatomical structures like the liver. The Chinese liver is defined by its functions, the Western liver by its physical structure.[1]

However, although they may reflect two different worlds, both treat the same conditions. In China the relevance of both disciplines in health care is accepted and they operate alongside each other in all major medical institutions. It is interesting to note that Chinese physicians of old were paid when the patient was well, but received no payment when he or she developed any form of disease. To quote the *Nei Ching*: 'The ancient sage did not treat those who were already ill; they instructed those who were not ill.'[2] And: 'The superior physician helps before the early budding of disease. The inferior physician begins to help when the disease has already developed; he helps when destruction has already set in. And since his help comes when disease has already developed, it is said of him that he is ignorant.'[3]

The *Nei Ching* is widely referred to as the bible of Chinese medicine. The *Huang-di Nei-Ching* or the *Yellow Emperor's Classic of Internal Medicine*, the source of all Chinese medical theory, is considered the equivalent of the *Corpus Hippocraticum* which originated at about the same time. It is the oldest of the Chinese medical texts, dating back about 4500 years. *The Classic of Internal Medicine* was supposed to have been written by the Yellow Emperor Huang To (2697–2596 BC) who reigned in China in about 2600 BC. The book describes conversations between the Yellow Emperor and his royal physician, Chi Po. Given the complexity of the Chinese language, translation of this work has been difficult. The quotations used in this particular book are derived mainly from the 1972 edition of the translation by Dr Ilza Veith of California University

Traditional Chinese medicine, which still adheres largely to the old wisdom, incorporates acupuncture, diet, manipulation and massage, hydrotherapy, herbalism, sun and air therapy, and exercise. Developed over thousands of years, it is deeply rooted in philosophy and has its own unique perception of physiology, health and disease. The realm of Chinese medicine is vast and complex and it is not necessary to become an absolute authority on this system in order to incorporate some of its knowledge and wisdom

into the realm of reflexology. It is also not the object of this book to elucidate on Chinese medicine in profound depth. But in order to include meridian therapy with reflexology, it is necessary to understand the relationship between the meridians and reflexology as well as to grasp certain important concepts of Chinese medical philosophy—most notably the theory of Yin and Yang, the five Elements, and the meridians themselves.

TAOISM

The philosophy of Taoism plays a central role in the formulation of Chinese medicine, so it must be briefly mentioned. Taoism has existed in China for approximately 2600 years. The Tao is the Law which maintains and orders the entire universe and the Taoist principles prescribe a way of life which involves abiding by these laws in order to maintain perfect balance, health and long life.

No words can accurately describe the Tao. Lao Tzu, the Chinese philosopher and metaphysician who lived in the sixth century BC is reputedly the founder of Taoism. As the author of the *Tao Te Ching* – a political treatise and theoretical representation of Taoism – he says: '"Tao" is just a convenient term for what is Nameless: I do not know its name so I call it Tao. If you insist on a description, I may call it vast, active, moving in great cycles . . . "Nothingness" is the name for it prior to the universe's birth. "Being" is the name for it as the Mother of Myriad Objects. Therefore when you seek to comprehend its mystery, it is seen as an unending void; when you seek to behold its content, you see that it is being.'[4]

John Blofeld's description from his book *Taoism* is probably one of the most succinct definitions to come from a Westerner: 'The Tao is unknowable, vast, eternal. As undifferentiated void, pure spirit, it is the mother of the cosmos; as non-void, it is the container, the sustainer and in a sense, the being of the myriad objects, permeating all. As the goal of existence, it is the Way of Heaven, of Earth, of Man. No being, it is the source of Being. It is not conscious of activity, has no purpose, seeks no reward or praise, yet performs all things to perfection. Like water, it wins its way by softness. Like a deep ravine, it is shadowy rather than brilliant. As Lao Tzu taught, it is always best to leave things to the Tao, letting it take its natural course without interference; for, "the weakest thing in heaven and earth, it overcomes the strongest; proceeding from no place, it enters where there is no crack. Thus do I know the value of non-activity. Few are they who recognise the worth of teaching without words and of non-activity."'5

The Tao is manifest in all things through the dynamic interaction of the two complementary forces, yin and yang.

YIN AND YANG

Says the *Nei Ching*: 'The principle of yin and yang is the basis of the entire universe. It is the principle of everything in creation . . . Heaven was created by an accumulation of yang; the Earth was created by an accumulation of yin. . . Yin and yang are the source of power and the beginning of everything in creation. . . Yang ascends to heaven; Yin descends to earth. Hence the universe (heaven and earth) represents motion and rest controlled by the wisdom of nature. Nature grants the power to beget and to grow, to harvest and to store, to finish and to begin anew.'6

Yin is seen as negative, passive, female, interior, dark; yang as positive, active, male, exterior, light – or any other pair of complementary qualities. Earth and moon are associated with yin; sky and sun are associated with yang. This dualism is evident in all things in the universe.

Yin and yang are constantly interacting and changing and neither can exist in isolation from the other. Because all things in the universe are constantly changing, nothing is entirely yin or yang. The *Nei Ching* states, 'Yin is active within and is the guardian of the yang, whereas yang is the dominant force on the outside and it is the regulator of the yin.'7

The relationship between yang and yin is also incorporated into the physical structure of man. Their affinity to each other is believed to have a decisive influence upon man's health. Perfect harmony between these two elements means health; disharmony or the undue preponderance of one element brings disease and death.8

In terms of health and the Chinese Taoist medicine, the interplay of yin and yang exerts its influence on two energies – 'macrocosmic energy' (Li – yang), which is the energy of the universe, and 'internal energy' (ch'i – yin), which is the energy within the human body. Both of these can have a great influence on the good health of every individual.9

THE FIVE ELEMENTS

It is believed that yin and yang further subdivide into five elements: water, fire, metal, wood and earth. Man, as a product of heaven and earth by the interaction of yin and yang, therefore also contains the five elements.10 The five elements will be discussed in more depth later in this section.

CH'I

The concept of ch'i, an integral aspect of Chinese medicine, is not recognized by Western medical science due to the lack of sufficient scientific proof. To the Chinese the existence of ch'i has long been accepted as undisputed fact.

Ch'i – which is not visible to the naked eye – can be equated with some form of electric energy, imperative for the existence of life. This natural internal body energy is often referred to as 'vital energy', 'life force' or 'vital force'. It circulates throughout the body in a well-defined cycle along specific pathways known as meridians, which are discussed in depth in Chapter 2.

All the organs, muscles, blood vessels and cells are reliant on ch'i for function and performance. Ch'i and its flow are possibly associated with the autonomic nervous system, which is linked to every organ and to all parts of the anatomy, including the skin tissue and glands. When ch'i is stimulated or sedated, it is registered by the autonomic nervous system which in turn affects specific areas of the organs or various parts of the body.[11]

Everyone is born with ch'i, and it remains with us until we die. Studies have been conducted in which dying people have been put on a scale and weighed. At the point of death there has been a recorded weight loss of approximately six ounces – the exact amount varying from individual to individual. It seems that this weight loss could reflect the weight of the vital energy.[12] The maintenance of health is dependent on this energy flowing freely throughout the body to animate all the body structure.

Ch'i is constantly depleted through the pressures of daily living and must be correctly cultivated and maintained for healthy functioning. Ch'i is augmented by energy obtained from food and air. Bad eating and drinking habits, lifestyle and attitudes, and shallow breathing tendencies will disrupt and deplete this energy, causing disease.

Although ch'i cannot be seen, it is believed to have been measured through sensitive electromagnetic machines, and is said to have been photographed by infrared sensitive film. So many scientists in China are now concentrating their research on ch'i that a special branch of science has developed called chiconology.[13] This research is being conducted with the assistance of practitioners of Qi gong – an ancient practice that involves controlling the movement of ch'i around the body. Qi gong

practitioners can apparently concentrate ch'i and expel it out of their bodies, and are reputed to be healthy, strong and less susceptible to disease.

If all the natural processes of the body and the strength of the internal energy are balanced and harmonious, good health is inevitable. However, fluctuations and changes constantly occur within the whole system, which could result in imbalances or disturbances. If the internal energy is not sufficiently strong to maintain equilibrium between all the bodily functions, disease will be the result.[14]

Reflexology works to help attain and maintain the equilibrium in the ch'i by activating the sections of the meridians present on the feet. This is why it is important to incorporate the concept of meridian therapy with the practice of reflexology.

Chinese medicine is essentially holistic. It is based on the idea that disease cannot be isolated from the patient and that no single part can be understood except in its relation to the whole. Nothing is treated symptomatically. According to the *Nei Ching*: 'Illness is comparable to the root; good medical work is comparable to the topmost branch; if the root is not reached, the evil influences cannot be subjugated.'[15]

The Chinese believe that illness is precipitated by environmental factors, emotions and lifestyle. They were particularly aware of climatic factors as they realized that the harmonious balance of yin and yang could be upset by prolonged exposure to extreme climatic conditions. The harmful effects of damaging emotions such as anger, fear, jealousy, worry or grief were considered to be even more destructive. The connection between diet and health was also considered vital, with food being analysed in terms of yin and yang – the food's heating or cooling effect, and stimulating or sedating action – as opposed to its chemical structure.

Today we are once again beginning to learn what the Chinese realized thousands of years ago; that disease is mostly the result of wrong living – not living in accord with the natural laws of the universe. Ancient Chinese philosophy regarded the human organism as a miniature version of the universe and often referred to man as 'the small world'. Thus, man cannot be divorced from nature as he forms an organic part of it. Nature as macrocosm and man as microcosm obey the same laws.

Says the *Nei Ching*: 'Those who rebel against the basic rules of the universe sever their own roots and ruin their true selves. Yin and yang, the two principles in nature, and the four seasons are the beginning and the end of everything and they are also the cause of life and death. Those who disobey the laws of the universe will give rise to calamities and visitations, while those who follow the laws of the universe remain free from dangerous illness, and they are the ones who have obtained Tao, the Right Way.'[16]

CHAPTER ONE

The Five Elements

There are no miracles, only unknown laws.
SAINT AUGUSTINE

In ancient China, people understood the importance of nature. Many healing arts were based on knowledge and insight gleaned from nature. They realized that as nature around them went through natural processes of change, the same patterns would occur within man.

The Chinese established five basic elements that interact in a creative cycle to form all other substances. These elements are wood, fire, earth, metal and water. The five elements do not refer to material elements, but rather conditions or states. Each of these elements is associated with a variety of factors: for example, body organs, sense organs, body tissue, colours, emotions, seasons, climate, and more. All these associations indicate only the predominant element; nothing is wholly any one element to the exclusion of others. Everything in existence contains all five elements but one element so predominates that it is named accordingly.[1]

In acupuncture, the principles governing the elements are used for specific diagnosis. Precise knowledge and understanding of the elements assists in ascertaining which organs and meridians are affected, and thus which acupuncture points should be stimulated or sedated, depending on the action required. To an acupuncturist, understanding the cycles of the elements is therefore of vital importance. Although reflexology does not work on the same principles, utilizing needles on precise acupuncture points, some knowledge of the five elements can facilitate better understanding of a person's condition.

Each cycle passes from element to element in a process of continual creation. Each element is produced by and produces another – one cannot exist without all the others. The five elements are generated or destroyed according to a law of cyclical interaction: fire produces earth, earth produces metal, metal finds water, water produces wood and wood becomes fire. By substituting for each element a corresponding yin organ, for example, we see that the heart (fire) aids or reinforces the action of the spleen/pancreas (earth); the spleen/pancreas affects the lungs (metal); the lungs, the kidneys (water); the kidneys, the liver (wood), and the liver the

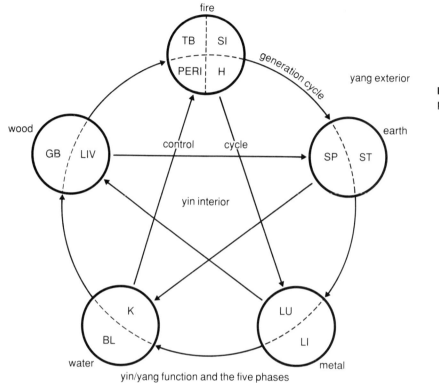

fire

TB | SI

PERI | H

generation cycle

yang exterior

wood

GB / LIV

control   cycle

earth

SP \ ST

yin interior

K

BL

LU

LI

water

metal

yin/yang function and the five phases

Fig. 80 Yin, yang and the five phases

heart. Conversely just as fire melts metal, metal cuts down wood, wood covers earth, earth absorbs water and water extinguishes fire, so the diseased or malfunctioning heart adversely affects the action of the lungs; the lungs affect the liver; the liver affects the spleen/pancreas, the spleen/pancreas affects the kidneys and the kidneys affect the heart.[2]

It is obvious how the nourishing and inhibiting cycle relates not only to the construction and working of the universe, but to the human body as well. This sequence is also evident in a psychological/physiological sense. The mind fuels the body with negative or positive thoughts. Negative thoughts breed destructive elements. Destructive elements create tension

and constrictions of circulation. Disease manifests in tense, sluggish areas of the body. The organs become diseased and fail to function. Our thinking becomes even more disturbed and negative. Pain permeates most of our days which causes us to become more and more dissociated from nature. Our vital energy becomes weaker and weaker. We die and go back to the earth.[3]

Although the stomach is referred to as an earth organ, and the kidneys a water organ, remember that these inner organs are classified according to element dominance. All organs have traces of the four others and it is through these traces that an organ is linked with other organs of a different element and the element's 'pool'. For example, the metal organs, lungs and large intestine, are linked through their water element trace with the water organs, kidneys and bladder; or through their wood element trace with the wood organs, liver and gall bladder. [4]

Each element is associated with inner organs – these are divided into two classes. The first are the six organs whose function is nutrition and excretion: stomach, large intestine, bladder, gall bladder, small intestine and the triple burner. The other six organs are associated with energy circulation, storage and distribution: spleen/pancreas, lungs, kidneys, liver, heart and circulation/pericardium. (The triple burner and circulation/pericardium are not actual organs in the sense of Western physiology, but fall into this category in Chinese medicine.) Apart from the organs, each element is identified with numerous other correspondences. Careful study of these will clarify their aid as diagnostic tools. Information on the corresponding organs and meridians is discussed in the chapter on meridians. In this section we will look briefly at symbolic parallels, and some of the more obvious, easy-to-read correspondences that can aid in diagnosis. These include season, climate, taste, colour, emotion and sound. Any extreme reactions to any of these factors (for example, either a strong aversion to or increased desire for any specific colour, season or taste) can indicate an imbalance in the related element.

The Chinese believed that climate had a profound effect on ch'i. Weather has a marked effect on the frequency of the meridians and a role in how the body copes with the various energies. Weather affects our lives, sometimes beneficially, often disruptively. We adapt to our environments to a certain extent, but any sudden change in climate can cause an imbalance. Any external forces experienced in excess can cause illness – which is why it is important to take special care of health at times of season change. An adverse reaction to, or preference for, a specific climate or season is important in traditional diagnosis. [5]

Emotion is also important. In a healthy state the human being should be able to feel and express all of the five emotions and their variations as it is appropriate. Every illness or imbalance is bound up with an emotion. [6] Sound is related to emotion. This can be perceived as a subtle tone in a person's voice or a vociferous expression of emotion, like shouting in anger or crying. Excessive or deficient emotion or sound can be correlated with a specific energy imbalance, depending on which type of emotion is being expressed.

Concerning the correspondence of taste, each flavour has an effect on energy. The combination of the five tastes ensures balance. An excess of one flavour can have an injurious effect, yet each element can be strengthened if the right flavour is prescribed for it. [7] The *Nei Ching* states: 'If people pay attention to the five flavours and blend them well, their bones will remain straight, their muscles will remain tender and young, breath and blood will circulate freely, the pores will be in fine texture, and consequently breath and bones will be filled with the essence of life.' [8] Any aversion to or obsession with a specific taste will indicate an imbalance in the related element.

The same applies to colour. A specific colour preference or dislike can provide useful information regarding element balance. Colour can also be perceived in the face. If ch'i is flowing harmoniously within each element and among the elements, the face will not show any predominant colour. If one of the elements is imbalanced, the colour associated with it will show, usually very clearly, on the face. This is not skin colour, but rather a subtle hue coming from the face. It is very real and has been used for thousands of years as one of the diagnostic tools in Chinese medicine. [9]

Other element correspondences relating specifically to body functions – sense organs, fluid secretions, orifice, part of body governed and external physical manifestation – are closely related to organ function. Any disturbances related to these correspondences clearly indicate specific energy imbalances within a particular element. The elements and some of their correspondences are discussed briefly here.

WOOD

Season Spring
Climate Wind
Organs Liver, gall bladder
Orifices Eyes
Sense organ Eyes
Body parts/tissue Muscles, sinews
Fluid secretion Tears
Physical manifestations Nails, hands, feet
Emotion Anger
Sound Shouting
Flavour Sour
Colour Green

Spring is the time for birth – for the human being to come alive, to be infused with the vital ch'i energy, to grow, to be reborn. In spring we sow the seeds for the autumn harvest within ourselves. If the healing seeds are not sown in the proper season, the person will not thrive.[10]

The wood element relates to spring – a time of generation of new life and the ability to be creative and capable of change. A well-rooted tree is strong and flexible, yielding to external pressures. It starts life as a small seed, blossoms into a sapling and develops into a mature and beautiful specimen which produces the seeds that contain the germ of new life. The description of a tree can be equated with a person. A healthy, well-rooted person will move effortlessly through the cycles of life. A strong wood element is evident in a flexible approach to life – a person will not become uprooted when confronted by life's pressures. This type of person is able to make complex life decisions,

plan ahead and execute the plans efficiently. When an idea takes root in a person with a strong wood element, it will germinate and bear fruit.[11]

When disturbed, the wood element can give rise to feelings of being emotionally stuck and to constriction, with tightness in the diaphragm, chest and throat.[12] It could also manifest physically as being off-balance and uprooted, easily confused and lacking ability to create roots for oneself. If wood is not sufficiently nourished and lacking in sunlight, it will lose its vitality. Insufficient wood element could also cause spinal problems, problems with articulation of the limbs, flexibility of movement and rootedness of the entire being.[13]

On the emotional level, balance in this element produces patience and good spirits. An imbalance results in aggression, difficulty in calming one's anger and the tendency to hit out in rage at anything in one's reach. Everyone gets angry at times, but if this condition is continuous it is more than likely an imbalance in the wood element. Aggression is also often a sign of imbalance in the gall bladder meridian which runs through the scalp and probably has a connection with the hypothalamus which is the centre of aggression. Problems with the liver, gall bladder, muscles, tendons, sinews, eyes, nails, hands and feet are related to this element.

FIRE

Season Summer
Climate Heat
Organs Heart, small intestine, circulation/
    pericardium and triple burner meridians
Orifices Ears
Sense organ Tongue
Body parts/tissue Blood vessels
Fluid secretion Perspiration
Physical manifestations Complexion
Emotion Joy, happiness

Sound Laughing
Flavour Bitter
Colour Red

The fire element relates to summer – the climate, warm. In nature things come to fruition in summer; so too in man. The sun warms our bodies and activates the growth process in plants. This element is the most yang. It is specifically in summer that problems in the fire element arise.

Fire is an active life principle. A good fire is dynamic and produces warmth and light. The energy on which a fire thrives is derived from wood. The fire element refers to all that is dynamic, vibrant and changing. A person with a strong fire element will be warm and caring and capable of great enthusiasm and excitement. A deficiency in the fire element, on the other hand, may show up as lack of enthusiasm or an inability to generate warmth for others. Lacking the energy to embrace life fully, such a person may have great difficulty becoming excited about anything.[14]

Emotionally, the fire element relates to love, happiness, gentleness and forgiveness. The element stimulates both physical body warmth and psychological warmth in our relationships with others. Lack of concern and love for others, as well as lack of energy to love oneself, is indicative of an imbalance on the emotional plane. One may also find it very difficult to forgive. These are signs of fire on the verge of burning out and can develop into emotional coldness, resulting in sexual frigidity, impotence, hysteria and total disinterest in closeness with others. Fire can also burn too furiously and this will manifest in excessive laughter, garrulous tendencies and overexcited, gesticulative behaviour. fire problems range from fever to frigidity. Heart, small intestine, ear and perspiration problems as well as speech impediments and complexion are related to this element.

EARTH

Season Late summer
Climate Dampness or humidity
Organs Spleen/pancreas, stomach
Orifices Mouth
Sense organ Mouth
Body parts/tissue Flesh, body shape
Fluid secretion Saliva
Physical manifestation Flesh
Emotion Sympathy
Sound Singing
Flavour Sweet
Colour Yellow

The season ruled by the earth element is late summer – not actually a season but a specific time of year. In old texts this season was said to be the last ten days of each of the four seasons and so a combination of them all.[15] This season falls in the middle of the year and is therefore very central and to a certain degree rules the other four elements. The earth element is often depicted outside the ordinary yin/yang divisions and is interpreted as harmony.

Earth is special among the elements because all the other elements derive their source from the earth, thus the earth is the central element for human life. Mother Earth provides us with life, support and nourishment. Food which nourishes us is grown in the earth. When we die, our physical bodies return to the earth. The earth holds water – the rivers and seas; contains metal in the minerals and rocks, and nourishes wood in the trees and plant life. The yin/yang within the earth element is influenced by the waxing and waning of the moon and the seasons.

The earth element refers not only to the ground on which we stand, but also to a sense of being grounded and rooted within ourselves. A person with a strong earth element will be centred, well-integrated and feel at home with him or herself as well as the outside world, at ease in all situations. A person suffering from a deficiency in this function may tend to become obsessed, constantly looking elsewhere for answers and support, and never realize that this must come from his or her own centre.[16] Emotionally, the earth element depicts sympathy and understanding. If one loses touch with the earth connection, self-pity, scepticism and cynicism can result.

Earth is the source of all physical nourishment, so anything involved with the intake of nourishment is connected to this element. The body thrives on the correct nourishment. Without this it will wither and die, and numerous diseases can be directly connected with poor nourishment. Thus, incorrect diet directly affects the earth – the centre. If the centre is deficient, it will inevitably affect the rest of the organism. The mouth and saliva are closely connected to the nourishment cycle, as it is in the mouth, through the action of the saliva, that the digestive process begins. And the physical manifestation, flesh, is also indicative of nutrition.

If the earth is off balance, all cycles lose their patterns – sleeping, breathing, thought processes, body harmony and coordination. Signs of distress in the earth element manifest in nervousness, instability, disconnectedness, insecurity. Problems with conception, sterility and birth can occur when the earth element is not sufficiently fertile. If the earth element is not correctly nourished in the parents, the children will suffer. A seed planted in deficient soil will have difficulty taking root, growing and coming to fruition; the fruit will be nutritionally deprived. If we care for ourselves, our children will be healthy and strong.[17]

METAL

Season Autumn
Climate Dry
Organs Lungs, large intestine

Orifices Nose
Sense organ Nose
Body parts/tissue Skin, body hair
Fluid secretion Mucus
Physical manifestation Skin, body hair
Emotion Melancholy
Sound Crying
Flavour Pungent
Colour White

The metal element relates to autumn – a time of slowing down, of harvesting and preparing for winter. It is a time when all things begin to conserve and store nourishment while externally life seems to be fading. As this is true in nature, it is also true in ourselves. If a person cannot harvest and store within themselves the things that are nourishing, that will carry them through the period of austerity, the body and mind will suffer. Maturity or harvesting the life experience is also associated with metal. Problems in the metal element relate to an inability to harvest and store one's own energy.[18]

The metal element can be associated with substance, strength and structure. It provides the main ingredient in systems of communication, provides substance with which to build communications and conducts electricity.[19]

In the human body, the ability to take in food and air, to assimilate and utilize fuel, and then to let go of unnecessary things are some life-sustaining aspects of the metal element. Problems with the structure and strength of the body and mind are symptoms of metal imbalance.[20] Emotionally, if energy is circulating as it should, one would feel positive and happy. If not, the opposite symptoms – depression, grieving and tendency to weep – will occur.

A person who is weak in the metal element will be slow and lethargic, will tend towards depression and lowered resistance – especially in autumn when he or she will suffer severe colds, influenza or bronchial problems. There will also be a tendency towards a general breakdown in communications, physically and emotionally. When metal is especially weak a more complex disturbance will occur, resulting from the inability of metal to control wood (liver and gall bladder functions) along the control cycle of the five elements. This may produce a feeling of weakness and pressure in the chest and tightness in the pit of the stomach (diaphragm) and an inability to muster the energy necessary to carry out life's plans.[21]

Any problems with the related organs, skin and body hair, point to a metal imbalance.

WATER

Season Winter
Climate Cold
Organs Kidneys, bladder
Orifices Genitals, urethra, anus
Sense organ Ears
Body parts/tissue Bones, bone marrow
Fluid secretion Saliva
Physical Manifestation Head hair
Emotion Fear
Sound Groaning
Flavour Salty
Colour Blue

The water element is related to winter, when all differences are evened out under a thick layer of snow. It is a time when nature hibernates, and conserves energy to enable herself to build up new resources. This element is the most yin. Warmth and nutrition are important at this time.

Water is essential to life. It is pliable yet extremely powerful. Water has a refreshing, invigorating quality. The human body is composed of approximately 75 per cent water, so without water human life would be impossible. The key words related to this element are *fluidity* and *flow*. Within the body, fluid must flow freely for efficient body functioning – blood flow, lymphatic secretions, urinary and endocrine fluidity, perspiration, tears and sexual secretions. All are influenced by the water element.[22]

Emotionally, the water element relates to self-confidence, courage and vitality. Lack of self-confidence, fear, tiredness, lack of energy and vitality are indicative of depleted energy in this element. Fear has its place in certain critical situations but if constant, it has a seriously debilitating effect. Lack of vitality in this element can also result in sexual and fertility problems. The water element is also the source of will-power, so a person with a disturbance here will lack the force necessary to accomplish or achieve anything in life. A deficiency in the water element will lead to a lifelong battle with fatigue, both physical and spiritual; a person with a severe deficiency will feel destined never to live fully and may be haunted by the spectre of serious illness. Such a person will often have gradually debilitating diseases.[23]

Fear and all kinds of phobias are related to this element. Fear can be thought of as holding on to rather than letting go of things that we feel anxious about. If energy is flowing well, we experience life like the flow of a river; if not, life is experienced like a nightmare, feeling overwhelmed and sinking into despair.[24]

Problems with related organs and body parts can be connected to the water element.

CHAPTER TWO

Meridians

Because the eye gazes but can catch no glimpse of it,
it is called elusive.
Because the ear listens but cannot hear it,
it is called rarefied.
Because the hand feels for it but cannot find it,
it is called the infinitesimal.
Its rising brings no light;
Its sinking no darkness.
It is called Ch'i.

TAO TE CHING

The Chinese believe that the vital life energy – ch'i – circulates in the body along meridians which are similar to the blood, nerve and lymphatic circuits. This vital life force controls the workings of all the systems of the body and in a truly healthy person will permeate all the cells. For each organ to maintain a state of perfect health, the ch'i must be able to flow freely along the meridians. The meridian system unifies all parts of the body, and is essential for the maintenance of harmonious balance. The *Nei Ching* says: 'The meridians move ch'i and blood, regulate yin and yang, moisten the tendons and bones, benefit the joints.' The meridian theory developed together with the evolution of acupuncture – a therapy that involves inserting fine needles into the skin at specific points. The

Chinese became aware that certain areas (points) were more sensitive when a body organ or function was impaired. These points seemed to form a definite path, a meridian, to the particular organ or function. Meridians form the basis of acupuncture, shiatsu and now, too, reflexology.

To the Chinese the meridians are an integral part of what makes us 'tick'. Although they have not been 'scientifically proven' to the satisfaction of orthodox medicine, tests are continuously undertaken in China to meet the demands for proof by the West. There are some theories worth considering.

An interesting discovery was made by a Japanese doctor, Dr Nagahama. While practising at a top Japanese university, he was treating a patient who had been struck by lightning and survived. The patient had extreme sensitivity of the skin as a result, and was able to describe pathways (quite unknown to him) on his body that seemed to be stimulated when the doctor inserted the needle in an acupuncture point. The paths the patient described were acupuncture meridians and *not* nervous pathways. Dr Nagahama then found that the speed of transmission along these meridians was entirely different from that along nerves (about ten times slower) and also confirmed that there were interconnections between meridians, as the Chinese had claimed for centuries.

Research to indicate the presence of the acupuncture points situated along the meridians has been relatively successful. Studies of acupuncture points show that they have extraordinary electrical properties. The points can be distinguished electrically from surrounding skin and also differ electrically from each other. The Russians developed an electronic machine called a tobiscope which flashes whenever it passes over an acupuncture point. A bright flash is said to show a healthy acupuncture point; a dull flash, potential or actual disease.[1]

According to John Thie of *Touch for Health* fame: 'Meridians contain a free-flowing, colourless, non-cellular liquid which may be partly actuated by the heart. These meridians have been measured and mapped by modern technological methods, electronically, thermally and radioactively. There are specific acupuncture points along the meridians. These points are electro-magnetic in character and consist of small oval cells called Bonham Corpuscles which surround the capillaries in the skin, the blood vessels and the organs throughout the body. There are some five hundred points which are most frequently used. They are stimulated in a definite sequence depending on the action required.'[2]

Ch'i circulates through the entire body within a twenty-four hour period. Each organ has a two-hour minimum period of activity and a two-hour minimum period of flow. If ch'i is slowed down or restricted by some internal blockage, or is made to flow faster than normal through an external influence, or there is extra energy in the system, then the body is thrown out of balance and this can result in sickness.[3]

There is actually only one continuous meridian which traverses the entire body, but this is divided into fourteen sections which are described according to their positions and functions. Of the fourteen meridians, twelve are considered the 'main' meridians. These are bilateral (paired), giving twenty-four separate pathways. Each meridian is connected and related to a specific organ from which it gets its name – in most cases the organs are those we are familiar with. It is also connected to a coupled meridian and organ with which it has a specific relationship. The coupled meridians consist of a yin and yang aspect, and come under the dominance of one of the five elements; for example, the kidney (yin) meridian is related to the bladder (yang) meridian and they are both ruled by the water element.[4]

The two extra meridians are known as the governing vessel and the conception vessel and run along the centre of the body – the conception vessel along the front and the governing vessel along the back.

It is difficult to draw a dividing line between the anatomical and physiological concepts of the *Nei Ching*. The organs are described for their function rather than for their location and structure, and the idea of cosmology, in other words the continuous interaction of yin and yang, the four seasons and the five elements, dominates the theories on structure as well as those on function.[5]

According to the *Nei Ching* man has five 'viscera' and six 'bowels'. The viscera, which are yin, are the heart, spleen, lungs, liver and kidneys. These have the capacity of storing but not of elimination. They determine the function of all the other parts of the body, including the 'bowels', and also of the spiritual resources and emotions.[6] The function of yin organs is to produce, transform, regulate and store the fundamental substances – ch'i, blood, jing, shen (spirit) and body fluids.[7] Jing is best translated as 'essence'. It is the substance that underlies all organic life. It is the source of organic change, and is generally thought of as fluid-like. Jing is supportive and nutritive and is the basis of reproduction and development.[8]

Digestion was held to be caused by the collaboration of yin and yang and the five viscera in the following manner: the food enters the stomach; its essence flows into the liver and from there its vital forces go into the muscles, its putrid gases ascend to the heart and its essence reaches the pulse, and finally its bulk descends by way of the anus. Drink enters the stomach and then turns into secretion, the essence of which enters the spleen. The spleen in turn sends its secretions to the lungs from which they descend to the bladder.[9]

The six 'bowels' are yang organs and have the capacity of elimination but not of storing. These are the gall bladder, stomach, large intestine, small intestine, bladder and the triple burner – or three burning spaces.[10] This is not an actual organ, and will be discussed in more depth in the detailed description of meridians. The yang organs receive, break down and absorb that part of the food that will be transformed into fundamental substances, and transport and excrete unused portions.[11]

The position of the viscera and bowels is compared to that of various officials in an empire, of which there are twelve, relating to the twelve main organs and meridians. The twelve officals must always work together for the maintenance of the whole, and never fail to assist one another. 'When the monarch is intelligent and enlightened, there is peace and contentment among his

subjects; thus they can beget offspring, bring up their children, earn a living, and lead a long and happy life. And because there are no more dangers and perils, the earth is considered glorious and prosperous.'[12]

THE MERIDIAN CYCLE

Meridians are classified yin or yang on the basis of the direction in which they flow on the surface of the body. The six yang meridians flow along the lateral aspect of the arms and legs, the face and the back, while the yin meridians flow along the inner aspect of the arms and legs and the pelvic and thoracic regions. If the human body were depicted on all fours, the aspects of the body's surface exposed to the sun (yang) would constitute the pathways of the yang meridians, while the aspect open to the earth (yin) would constitute the yin meridians..

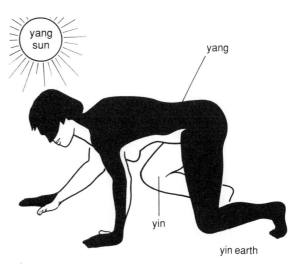

Fig. 81 Yin and yang on the human body

Meridians interconnect deep within the torso and have an internal branch and a surface branch. The section which is worked on is the surface branch which is accessible to touch techniques. Yang energy flows from the sun, and yang meridians run from the fingers to the face, or from the face to the feet. Yin energy from the earth flows from the feet to the torso and from the torso along the inside (yin side) of the arms to the fingertips. Since this is actually one continuous unbroken flow, the energy moves in a definite direction and from one meridian to another in a well-determined order. As there is no beginning or end to this flow, the order of the meridians is represented as a wheel which follows this order in the body:

- From torso to fingertips – along the inside of the arm = yin.

- From fingertips to face – along the outside/back of the arm = yang.

- From face to feet – along the outside of the leg = yang.

- From feet to torso – along the inside of the leg = yin.[13]

THE CHINESE CLOCK/MIDDAY–MIDNIGHT LAW

The Chinese recognized a 24-hour movement of energy, referred to as the Chinese Clock. This 'clock' is a 24-hour cycle which divides the day and night into two-hour periods. Each one of

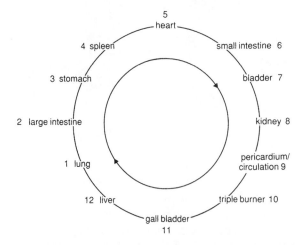

Fig. 82 Order of energy flow through the meridians

these is associated with a surge of energy in one of the organs and its meridian. For example, between the hours of 3 and 5 am, the lungs receive their daily booster. The cycle begins with the lungs and for this reason it is said that these are the hours when it is most suitable to be born.[14]

The Chinese also believe that the best time for stimulating a particular organ is at the appropriate two-hour period when its energy is 'full'. Alternatively it should be sedated at the opposite period of the day or night. For example, the lungs should be stimulated between 3 and 5 am and sedated between 3 and 5 pm. The organ maximum energy periods are included in the detailed section on meridians.[15]

MERIDIANS AND REFLEXOLOGY

The concept of energy channels is the central point around which the practices of reflexology and acupuncture are based. Both function on the premise that vital energy is channelled throughout the body along specific pathways. In acupuncture, these energy lines are the meridians. In reflexology, as has been perceived to date, the energy channels are those of the zones popularized by Dr W. Fitzgerald.

Both practices assert that disease is caused by blockages in energy channels. The acupuncture points, situated all over the body, are stimulated or sedated usually with needles. Reflexology concentrates only on the feet, stimulating with specific finger pressure techniques the reflex areas as well as the sections of meridians situated here.

Think of meridians as electrical pathways. If molecules become congested along parts of the pathway, it can cause pain. With acupuncture, reflexology or any other therapy that works on the energy forces of the body, the practitioner exerts a force which causes the molecules to disperse, thereby allowing the energy to flow freely again. Close study of the meridians reveals that the six main meridians – those that penetrate the major body organs – are represented in the feet, specifically in the toes. Thus, massaging the feet helps clear congestions in the meridians. Meridians theory assumes that a disorder within a meridian generates derangement in the pathway and creates disharmony along that meridian, or that such derangement is a result of a disharmony of the meridian's connecting organ. A disorder in the stomach meridian, for example, may cause upper toothache because the meridian passes through the upper gums, while lower toothache may be the result of a disorder of the large intestine meridian. Pain in the groin may as easily result from a liver meridian disorder as from a disorder of the liver itself.[16]

A knowledge of meridians can help reflexologists to more comprehensively understand the disease pathway. A basic knowledge of meridians can be of enormous benefit in pinpointing problem areas. If, for example, pain, irritation or any other condition does not improve satisfactorily through treatment of the reflex area, one should observe the meridian which traverses the part of the body in question, and treat the reflex area of the organ related to that particular meridian.

The meridians can be used simply and effectively for a better understanding of conditions. Take, for example, a person with arthritis in the little finger, tennis elbow, fibrositis in the shoulder blade, infection in the lymph glands of the throat, trigeminal neuralgia and hearing problems. One need simply look at the small intestine meridian – this starts in the little finger, ends just in front of the ear and passes the locations of all the above disorders. Could this mean that the small intestine disorder could aggravate or even cause these problems? Clinical results of balancing the meridians indicate this.

If a person is suffering from pain in the right knee, question exactly where the pain is situated

– on the front, back, inner or outer section of the knee. If the pain is on the outer side, it will fall into the gall bladder meridian. The gall bladder reflex should then be treated, and will usually be found to be sensitive. Although the organ itself may not be diseased, the congestion on the meridian is causing pain and discomfort.

It is important to distinguish between 'organ conditions' and 'energy conditions'. An 'organ condition' is evident when an organ is not functioning properly. This could manifest as digestive or respiratory problems, hormonal disturbances and the like. 'Energy conditions' – like headaches, sciatica, trigeminal neuralgia and hip pains – are more difficult to define. These conditions are often found along a meridian pathway, and the related organ reflex will usually be sensitive. This does not necessarily indicate an organ disorder. Energy conditions are usually forerunners of more serious problems, and if they are not treated early on, they can eventually influence the related organ and result in a chronic problem. (See Figure 83.)

Pains in the fingers and toes often indicate which meridian is congested. For example, pains in the index finger refer to the large intestine meridian, while pains in the big toe could refer to either the liver or spleen/pancreas meridians. (See Figure 84.)

SYMPTOMS/SIGNS TO NOTE ALONG MERIDIANS

Before we look into the meridians in more depth, we must briefly discuss certain common and obvious disorders which indicate congestions and where these may be situated. These disorders may take the form of skin conditions, warts, birthmarks, lumps, nail problems and the like.

If a person has skin problems, it may be that the lungs and large intestine are the root cause. But note must be taken of exactly where the

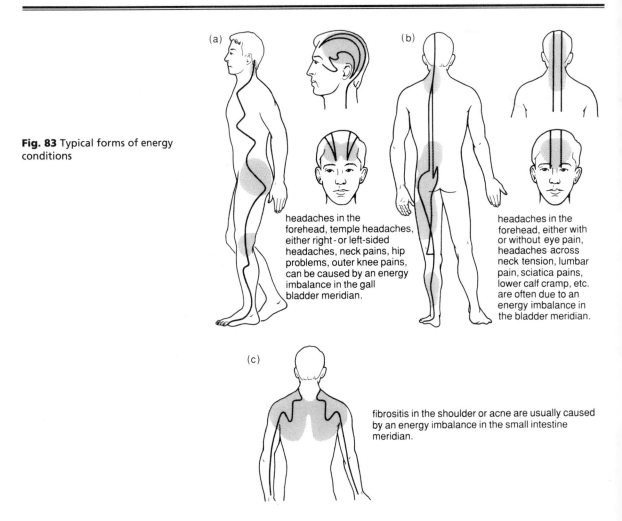

Fig. 83 Typical forms of energy conditions

headaches in the forehead, temple headaches, either right- or left-sided headaches, neck pains, hip problems, outer knee pains, can be caused by an energy imbalance in the gall bladder meridian.

headaches in the forehead, either with or without eye pain, headaches across neck tension, lumbar pain, sciatica pains, lower calf cramp, etc. are often due to an energy imbalance in the bladder meridian.

fibrositis in the shoulder or acne are usually caused by an energy imbalance in the small intestine meridian.

problem manifests on the body. Often these will occur parallel to each other – someone with psoriasis may have it on the outer side of the leg (gall bladder meridian) and down the back (bladder meridian).

Check the nails for white spots, whitlows, ridges, problems with the roots of the nail or any other defects. Ridges often indicate high acidity. If you note on which meridian the problem manifests, it will be obvious where the congestion is placed. If it is on the thumb, acidity is congesting the lung meridian. If there are white spots on the nails, these indicate deficiency. As the nail takes approximately three

months to grow, by dividing the nail into segments one will be able to see the approximate period when the deficiency occurred, and relate it to the situation at the time. For example, the person may have been on a sugar binge or through a great deal of stress which could have caused the deficiency. Always note these signs and pinpoint the meridian on which they appear in order to trace where the problems may lie.

Muscles

Muscular symptoms are also extremely important and revealing in relating problems to causes.

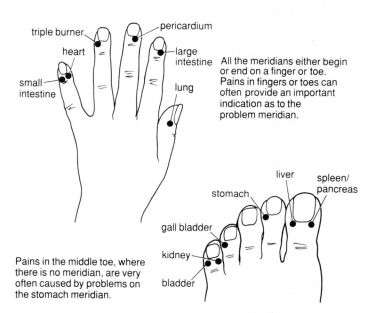

triple burner
pericardium
heart
large intestine
small intestine
lung

All the meridians either begin or end on a finger or toe. Pains in fingers or toes can often provide an important indication as to the problem meridian.

Fig. 84 Correspondences between meridians, toes and fingers

liver
spleen/pancreas
stomach
gall bladder
kidney
bladder

Pains in the middle toe, where there is no meridian, are very often caused by problems on the stomach meridian.

Muscular problems are often the main reason many people seek assistance and treatment. The muscles also relate to specific meridians and organs, and understanding this relationship can enable you to assist the deficient organ back to an optimum state of health, thereby eliminating muscle problems.

The muscles form the flesh of the body. There are two types of muscle: *voluntary* muscle, made up of striped or cross-banded tissue, and *involuntary* muscle comprising smooth cells without cross stripes.

Each voluntary muscle consists of a large number of separate fibres. These are bound together in bundles by a sheath of connective tissue called the *perimysium*. The whole muscle is then covered by a sheet of fibrous tissue called *fascia*, and is connected to the bone by tendons.

When stimulated, each muscle fibre contracts – gets shorter and thicker. As the muscle passes over one or more joints, this contraction will pull one bone towards the other, thus producing movement at the joint. The type of movement depends on the position and shape of the muscles and the type of joint they cross. A muscle must

have an adequate blood and nerve supply before it can contract. It receives glucose and oxygen from the blood. The nerve supplies the impulse which starts off a series of chemical changes involving glucose and oxygen. These changes release the energy which makes the muscles contract.[17]

When movement is required, carbohydrates are broken down, oxygen is carried to muscles in the bloodstream and a series of chemical changes occur which release energy and produce heat. The energy makes the muscle contract and the heat helps to keep the body temperature at 37°C. The waste produced by muscle action is carbon dioxide and water, which are conveyed by the blood to the lungs and breathed out, although some of the water is also excreted by the skin, the bladder and the bowel. The muscles become inactive if anything interferes with the blood and nerve supply.

The relationship between muscles and meridians was accidentally discovered in the 1960s by a chiropractor from Detroit, Dr George Goodheart. This practice is today known as 'Applied Kinesiology' and shares the basic premises of acupuncture and shiatsu. Goodheart discovered that the tests used in kinesiology to determine the relative muscle strength and tone over the range of movement of the joints could also reveal the balance of energy in each of the body's systems. Further research led him to identify the relationship between each specific muscle group, the particular organs and the meridians of acupuncture.

The assumption used to be that the main muscular troublemakers in backache and associated disorders were muscles which were either in spasm or too taut, thus affecting the spine. Goodheart, however, began to work on a different idea; that it might not be the muscle spasm or tautness that was the problem, but rather that it was 'weak muscles' on the opposite side of the body which caused the normal muscles to appear 'tight'. Combining Eastern ideas about energy flow with his own chiropractic techniques, Goodheart developed his new system. Goodheart's original research is being expanded and more investigations are being carried out by many chiropractors who have found Applied Kinesiology of inestimable value as a diagnostic aid.

In reflexology we do not practise muscle testing to ascertain weakness in the body. This knowledge can, however, be useful to reflexologists. For example, a person with headaches on the bladder meridian, may also have weak eyes and suffer calf cramps. The calf muscles (soleus and gastrocnemius) are both related to the bladder and its meridian, confirming an imbalance. Another form of headache may be associated with the gall bladder meridian. The person may have related symptoms such as nausea, hip pain or a frozen shoulder. The shoulder muscle (anterior deltoid) is related to the gall bladder and its meridian.

I have also seen clients with weight problems who are unable to shed the weight from their thigh or calf muscles. The calf muscles (gastro-cnemius and soleus) and thigh muscles (sartorius and gracilis) are related to the triple burner (endocrine) meridian, thus indicating a hormonal imbalance as the cause of the weight problem. Muscle-related disorders associated with the kidney meridian are problems with the neck/shoulder area and the hip/pelvic area. Many people complain of neck tension and believe the cause to be merely tension. However, it could be the result of overloading the kidneys and bladder. If toxins are not efficiently eliminated by the kidneys, they may be stored in the neck or hip regions. If this is not corrected the toxins remain in these muscles and eventually begin to eat away at the bone structure.

It is thus obvious how muscle problems can indicate organ imbalance. This is further clarified by an interesting case history. A male in his early sixties had suffered a frozen shoulder for six months. His doctor offered little hope of improvement and the only relief he could give was cortisone injections. When he came for reflexology treatment, I enquired about the state of his gall bladder, and was informed that it had been removed during the war. The doctors had been puzzled at the time as the organ appeared quite healthy, apart from being slightly enlarged. The client then mentioned a 'souvenir' from the war – a bullet behind his knee – right in the area which relates to the gall bladder. This could well have been the cause of the frozen shoulder and the enlarged gall bladder! The muscles related to the meridians are illustrated in the detailed section on meridians.

LUNG MERIDIAN

Yin meridian
Partner meridian Large Intestine (Yang)
Element Metal.
Organ maximum energy period 3am to 5am

The *Nei Ching* states: 'The lungs are the symbol of the interpretation and conduct of the official

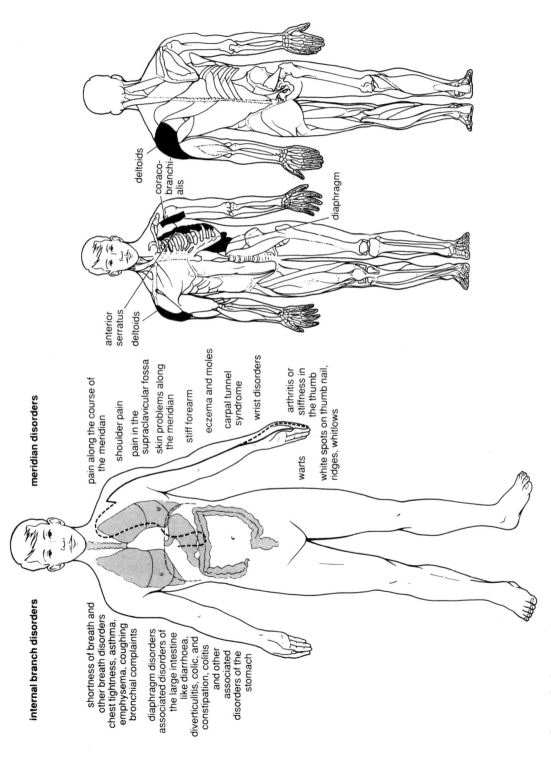

internal branch disorders

shortness of breath and other breath disorders chest tightness, asthma, emphysema, coughing bronchial complaints

diaphragm disorders associated disorders of the large intestine like diarrhoea, diverticulitis, colic, and constipation, colitis and other associated disorders of the stomach

meridian disorders

pain along the course of the meridian

shoulder pain

pain in the supraclavicular fossa

skin problems along the meridian

stiff forearm

eczema and moles

carpal tunnel syndrome

wrist disorders

arthritis or stiffness in the thumb

white spots on thumb nail, ridges, whitlows

warts

deltoids

coraco-branchi-alis

diaphragm

anterior serratus

deltoids

Fig. 85 The lung meridian and muscles associated with the lung meridian

jurisdiction and regulation'.[18] And, 'The lungs are the origin of the breath and the dwelling of the animal spirits or inferior soul. The lungs influence the body hair and have their effects upon the skin.'[19]

The lungs and large intestine are partner meridians and both govern elimination. The lungs excrete carbon dioxide, and the large intestines solid residue. Due to their close relationship, they can directly affect each other; for example, chest problems can be accompanied by constipation and diarrhoea, and vice versa.[20]

The lungs regulate respiration and are therefore responsible for the ch'i of the entire body. Ch'i from the air outside is inhaled into the lungs where it comes into contact with the ch'i inside the body. Healthy lungs and regular, even respiration ensure that ch'i enters and leaves the body smoothly. An imbalance in the function of this organ or meridian will result in various forms of chest problems.[21]

Respiratory functions affect all the rhythms of the body, including the blood flow. The lungs are also concerned with the movement and transformation of water in the body. They liquify water vapour and move it down to the kidneys. The secretion of sweat is regulated by the lungs, as they work to scatter water vapour throughout the body to be eliminated via the skin and pores. As the nose and throat are included in the respiratory functions, they too are related to the lungs. The lungs are referred to as the 'delicate organ' as they are most easily influenced by external environmental factors.[22]

The lung meridian has a descending flow of energy which runs from the chest to the hand.

The lung meridian starts at the clavicle and ends on the back of the thumb towards the index finger (see diagram).

Meridian Disorders

Pain along the course of the meridian; shoulder pain in the depression above the clavicle; stiff forearm; skin problems along the meridian; wrist disorders (carpal tunnel syndrome); arthritis or stiffness in the thumb; warts along the meridian or any problems occurring on the thumb and thumbnail like white spots, ridges, whitlow, eczema and moles.

Internal Branch Disorders

Shortness of breath and other breathing disorders; chest tightness; asthma; emphysema; coughing; bronchial complaints; diaphgram disorders; associated disorders of the large intestine like diarrhoea; constipation; colitis; diverticulitis; colic and associated disorders of the stomach.

Muscles Related to this Meridian

Serratus Anterior (Yin) This muscle draws the shoulder blade forward and raises the ribs. Weakness will make it difficult to push things forward with the arms straight, causing the shoulder blades to wing out in the back. It can also affect chest conditions and the diaphragm's ability to regulate breathing.[23]

Coracobrachialis (Yin) This works with the anterior deltoid in straightening the arm when it is held over the head and in flexing the shoulder with the elbow bent as in combing the hair. They are not usually found weak.[24]

Deltoids (Yin) This is the triangular muscle of the shoulder arising from the clavicle and scapula, with insertion into the humerus. It draws the arm away from the body, lifting the elbow. Weakness will make it difficult to raise the arm. Lung problems such as bronchitis, pleurisy, pneumonia, congestion and flu will usually affect the deltoid.[25]

Diaphragm (Yin) The diaphragm is a muscular dome-shaped partition separating the chest cavity from the abdominal cavity. It is the chief muscle used in breathing. A disturbance in the

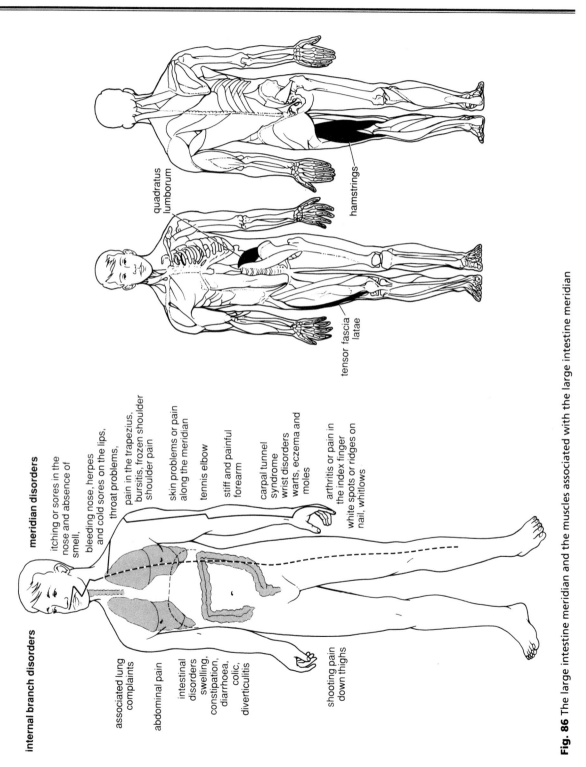

quadratus
lumborum

hamstrings

tensor fascia
latae

meridian disorders

itching or sores in the
nose and absence of
smell,

bleeding nose, herpes
and cold sores on the lips,
throat problems,

pain in the trapezius,
bursitis, frozen shoulder
shoulder pain

skin problems or pain
along the meridian

tennis elbow

stiff and painful
forearm

carpal tunnel
syndrome
wrist disorders
warts, eczema and
moles

arthritis or pain in
the index finger
white spots or ridges on
nail, whitlows

internal branch disorders

associated lung
complaints

abdominal pain

intestinal
disorders
swelling,
constipation,
diarrhoea,
colic,
diverticulitis

shooting pain
down thighs

Fig. 86 The large intestine meridian and the muscles associated with the large intestine meridian

muscle balance of the diaphragm can cause breathing difficulties, hiccups and reduce breath-holding time. There may be digestive disturbances, especially discomfort immediately after eating.[26]

LARGE INTESTINE MERIDIAN

Yang meridian
Partner meridian Lung (Yin)
Element Metal
Organ maximum energy period 5 am to 7 am

'The large intestines are like the officials who propagate the right way of living and they generate evolution and change,' states the *Nei Ching*.[27] As the 'generator of evolution and change', correct functioning of this organ is vital to the well-being of the whole body. The large intestine forms the lower part of the digestive tract and is in charge of transporting, transforming and eliminating surplus matter. The important function of elimination of waste material is imperative to the maintenance of health. If waste is not effectively excreted, the rest of the system has to cope with an additional load of toxins which will have a harmful effect on the entire system and cause disharmony throughout the body. Mental constipation – toxic thoughts and feelings – are often associated with this meridian, as well as physical constipation or diarrhoea.[28]

This meridian has an ascending flow of energy running from the hand to the head. It receives energy from the lung meridian and transmits it to the stomach meridian. The large intestine meridian starts on the back of the index finger, ascends up the arm and ends next to the nose (see diagram).

Meridian Disorders

Arthritis or pain in the index finger; any problems along index finger and nail including white spots, whitlows, ridges, warts; wrist disorders (carpal tunnel syndrome); stiff and painful forearm; tennis elbow; skin problems or pain along the meridian; shoulder pain; frozen shoulder; bursitis; pain in the trapezius muscle; throat problems; herpes/cold sores on the lips; and nose problems including bleeding, itching or sores in the nose and absence of smell.

Internal Branch Disorders

Associated lung complaints; intestinal disorders; abdominal pain, swelling, constipation, diarrhoea, colic, diverticulitis; shooting pain down the thighs.

Muscles Related to this Meridian

Tensor Fasciae Latae (Yang) This muscle helps flex or bend the thigh, draw it away from the body sideways, and keep it turned in. With weakness, the leg may tend to bow, the thigh turning outward.[29]

Hamstrings (Yang) These are situated in the back of the thigh. They flex the leg and turn the leg sideways when the knee is bent. Weakness will cause either a bow-legged or knock-kneed posture. Hamstrings are important in walking.[30]

Quadratus Lumborum (Yang) This flexes the vertebral column sideways, drawing it towards the hip. It assists in the action of the diaphragm in breathing. It is a major stabilizing muscle of the lower back. Weakness on one side of the muscle will show in the posture as an elevation of the last rib on the weak side and a curve in the lumbar vertebrae.[31]

STOMACH MERIDIAN

Yang meridian
Partner meridian Spleen/Pancreas (Yin)
Element Earth
Organ maximum energy period 7 am to 9 am

'The stomach acts as the official of the public granaries and grants the five tastes,' says the *Nei*

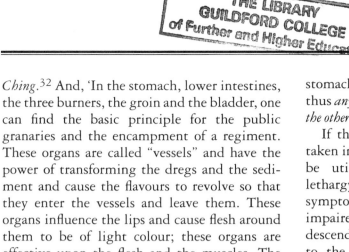
Ching.[32] And, 'In the stomach, lower intestines, the three burners, the groin and the bladder, one can find the basic principle for the public granaries and the encampment of a regiment. These organs are called "vessels" and have the power of transforming the dregs and the sediment and cause the flavours to revolve so that they enter the vessels and leave them. These organs influence the lips and cause flesh around them to be of light colour; these organs are effective upon the flesh and the muscles. The flavour connected with these organs is sweet and the colour is yellow.'[33]

The functions and activities of the stomach and spleen are closely related. The stomach controls digestion – it receives nourishment, integrates it and brings it to fruition and passes on the 'pure' food energy to be distributed by the spleen.[34] The spleen then transforms it into the raw material for ch'i and blood. If the stomach does not hold and digest food, the spleen cannot transform it and transport its essence. They are interdependent meridians. The directions of the ch'i activity complement each other – the spleen rules ascending and the stomach rules descending.[35]

According to Chinese philosophy the stomach is related to appetite, digestion and transport of food and fluids, but the partner meridian, the spleen/pancreas, is responsible for the ruling of food transport and energy consumption. The two meridians of the earth element work together more closely than any of the others to stabilize the individual. The earth element represents harmony and if there is no harmony in the stomach, spleen and pancreas, this will affect all the other organs.

The stomach is referred to as the 'sea of food and fluid' or 'sea of nourishment' as it governs digestion and is responsible for 'receiving' and 'ripening' ingested foods and fluids. Without the nourishing activities of the stomach, the other organs in the body could not function. The stomach is *central* physically and functionally; thus *any problem in the stomach is quickly reflected in the other organs.*

If this organ is out of balance, whatever is taken in, be it physical or psychic food, will not be utilized correctly. Energy depletion – lethargy, weakness and debilitation – are symptoms warning us that this function is impaired.[36] The stomach meridian has a descending flow of energy running from the head to the foot. It receives ch'i from the large intestine meridian and passes it on to the spleen meridian.

The stomach meridian starts under the eye and curves up to the temple. It then continues down the body and ends on the top of the second toe (see diagram).

Meridian Disorders

In this section, I am going to study the symptoms in some depth as I believe disharmony in the stomach to be the root cause of all disease in the body. The quality of the food ingested goes hand in hand with the quality of life you enjoy. If the fuel is faulty, the functions of the organs will be faulty and disease will be the ultimate result. The stomach meridian is the only meridian that penetrates all the major body organs.

We will begin with the section of the meridian that runs through the face. The internal stomach meridian and the bladder meridian meet at the inner corner of the eye. One could therefore conclude that imbalances in the stomach, such as excess acidity not eliminated via the kidneys and bladder, will manifest as eye weakness. Bags and shadows under the eyes are related to kidney disorders, even by the medical profession. The stomach meridian penetrates the kidneys. Another interesting phenomenon related to this area is the goitre which causes the eyes to bulge. Most medical doctors relate this specifically to thyroid problems, but if you take note of the path of the stomach meridian, you

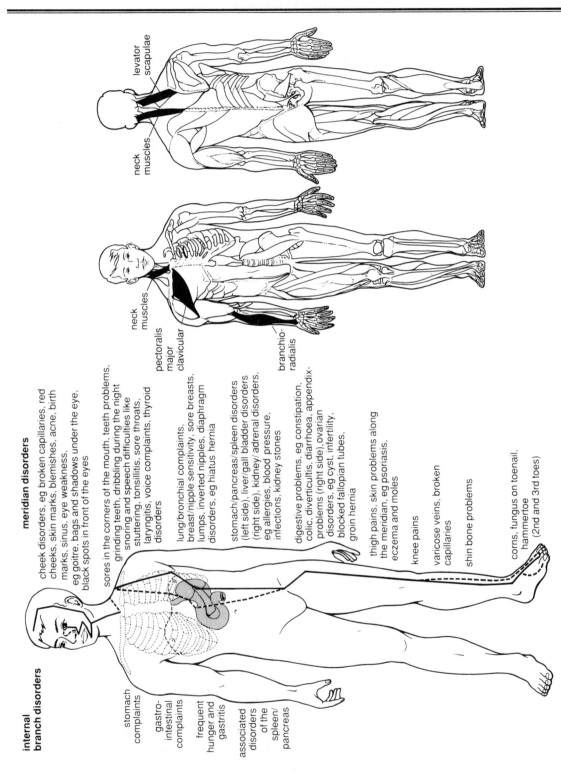

levator
scapulae

neck
muscles

neck
muscles

pectoralis
major
clavicular

branchio-
radialis

meridian disorders

cheek disorders, eg broken capillaries, red cheeks, skin marks, blemishes, acne, birth marks, sinus, eye weakness, eg goitre, bags and shadows under the eye, black spots in front of the eyes

sores in the corners of the mouth, teeth problems, grinding teeth, dribbling during the night snoring and speech difficulties like stuttering, tonsillitis, sore throats, laryngitis, voice complaints, thyroid disorders

lung/bronchial complaints, breast/nipple sensitivity, sore breasts, lumps, inverted nipples, diaphragm disorders, eg hiatus hernia

stomach/pancreas/spleen disorders (left side), liver/gall bladder disorders (right side), kidney/ adrenal disorders, eg allergies, blood pressure, infections, kidney stones

digestive problems, eg constipation, colic, diverticulitis, diarrhoea, appendix-problems (right side), ovarian disorders, eg cyst, infertility, blocked fallopian tubes, groin hernia

thigh pains, skin problems along the meridian, eg psoriasis, eczema and moles

knee pains

varicose veins, broken capillaries

shin bone problems

corns, fungus on toenail, hammertoe (2nd and 3rd toes)

**internal
branch disorders**

stomach
complaints

gastro-
intestinal
complaints

frequent
hunger and
gastritis

associated
disorders
of the
spleen/
pancreas

Fig. 87 The stomach meridian and the muscles associated with the stomach meridian

will notice that it runs directly through the thyroid, linking the stomach to the eyes. So again, the ultimate cause of this problem could be traced back to the stomach. This is also true of seeing black spots in front of the eyes, which are usually related to liver problems. But as the stomach meridian runs through the liver, the problem again can be traced back to the stomach. Squint eyes can be related to the stomach or bladder.

Sinus, sinus pain and hayfever also relate to the stomach meridian around the eye region. Broken capillaries in the cheeks and red cheeks can be indicative of bronchial problems like emphysema, spasms or lack of oxygen. The stomach meridian passes through this area as well. The meridian passes around the mouth area and problems here include sores in the corners of the mouth (which may be indicative of stomach or duodenal ulcers); split, cracked tongue which is a result of stomach acidity; problems with the teeth (specifically the molars), grinding teeth and dribbling during the night. If babies have severe teething and dribbling problems it would be advisable for mothers to look to the stomach as the cause, as teething problems are lessened if the stomach is well balanced. Teething problems often go hand in hand with nappy rash which is caused by high uric acid content, so a decrease in acidic food intake would help solve the problem.

Most skin problems can be traced back to a stomach imbalance. This is particularly true in females, whose facial skin problems are often tied in with their menstrual cycle. As the stomach meridian runs through the ovaries, problems will be accentuated during menstruation.

Many people are born with birthmarks on the face. If they look into their family background, they may discover a history of stomach complaints or a tendency to eat food of high acid content. Often during pregnancy, expectant mothers will develop a craving for acidic foods like oranges and chocolate, further upsetting the delicate acid/alkaline balance of the stomach. Contraceptive pills also upset this balance and often cause brown blemishes on the face. Although brown blemishes on the body are usually related to liver problems, the stomach meridian runs through the liver, and the stomach is more often than not the cause of upset in the liver.

Most throat problems can also be related to the stomach meridian as it passes through this area. Here you find problems such as tonsillitis, sore throats, laryngitis and voice complaints; thyroid problems which can cause metabolic disorders; snoring, and speech difficulties like stuttering.

From the throat, the meridian continues into the bronchial area, so imbalances here could result in various lung/bronchial complaints like bronchial spasm, emphysema, asthma, tight chest, mucus build-up, etc.

The meridian then runs through the nipple, and in women one will see complaints related to the menstrual cycle, such as sore breasts, inverted nipples, fibroids or cysts in the breasts. (There are in fact three meridians that pass through the breast, so if a cyst is the problem, one would have to locate the exact position in order to define the meridian on which it is situated.)

Below the breasts the meridian passes through the diaphragm so problems here, for example hiatus hernia, could be indicative of stomach disorders. The meridian runs through the liver/gall bladder on the right side of the body so complaints related to these organs could be caused by the stomach, while on the left side of the body, the meridian runs through the stomach, spleen, pancreas and duodenum. Problems such as ulcers, acid regurgitation, indigestion, blood sugar imbalance and appetite problems can be tied in here.

The meridian has a slight curve and enters the adrenals and kidneys on both sides. An imbalance in the adrenals and kidneys can often be linked to allergic problems, blood pressure disorders, bladder or kidney infections, kidney stones, oedema and heart problems. Again, the stomach meridian penetrates these organs and can be traced as the cause.

As the meridian descends, it enters the large and small intestines, affecting the digestion, can be related to problems like constipation, diarrhoea, diverticulitis and colic. Further down, the meridian runs through the appendix and ovaries, linking it to problems such as appendicitis, ovarian cysts, menstrual cycle complaints, infertility, blocked Fallopian tubes, etc. In the groin region, hernias often occur on the stomach meridian.

This meridian then runs down the thighs linking the stomach to thigh complaints, varicose veins and broken capillaries. Along the path of the meridian, skin problems like psoriasis, eczema and moles can occur. When the meridian reaches the knees, one must take careful note of exactly where the problem is, as six meridians run through the knees at different points. Further down, one will find associated disorders of the shin.

In the foot the meridian runs along the dorsal area and problems may be expressed in pains or problems like toenail fungus, corns, bent or malformed toes and the like, in the second and third toes, particularly the second. If the second toe is longer than the big toe, this indicates a genetic weakness in the stomach meridian. This does not necessarily mean the person will have problems in the stomach area. If their lifestyle is healthy, it is unlikely, but if not, they would be more prone than others to imbalances in the stomach and its meridian.

Then, of course, one must also consider the muscles related to the stomach – the neck and chest muscles. Problems here could be caused by excess acidity in the stomach.

Internal Branch Disorders

Stomach complaints – gastro-intestinal complaints, frequent hunger and gastritis, and associated disorders of the spleen/pancreas.

Muscles Related to this Meridian

Pectoralis Major (Clavicular) (Yang) This chest muscle helps turn the arm in at the shoulder. Treating the reflexes for this muscle affects both the stomach and the emotional centres within the brain.[37]

Levator Scapulae (Yang) These muscles in the back of the shoulders and neck are often found weak, causing the neck to twist with the head staying level. If there were persistent tension in this muscle, chiropractic adjustment of the neck may be necessary.[38]

Neck Muscles (Yang) These muscles are the anterior neck flexors in the front and sides of the neck. They can easily be affected by whiplash injuries, making it difficult to lift or turn the head. They are normally not quite as strong as the muscles in the back of the neck. If the muscles in the front become weak, the neck forms an 'S' curve causing the head to balance improperly on the spine. This can be the source of headaches and shoulder tension.[39]

Brachioradialis (Yang) This muscle flexes the elbow and helps turn the wrist. A weakness of this muscle may make it difficult to get the arm up and behind the back.[40]

SPLEEN/PANCREAS MERIDIAN

Yin meridian
Partner meridian Stomach (Yang)
Element Earth
Organ maximum energy period 9 am to 11 am

The *Nei Ching* states: 'The spleen rules transformation and transportation'.[41] It is the crucial link in the process by which food is transformed into ch'i and blood. If this process of food transformation is not activated, nourishment and ch'i are not available for important body functions. If the transformative and transporting

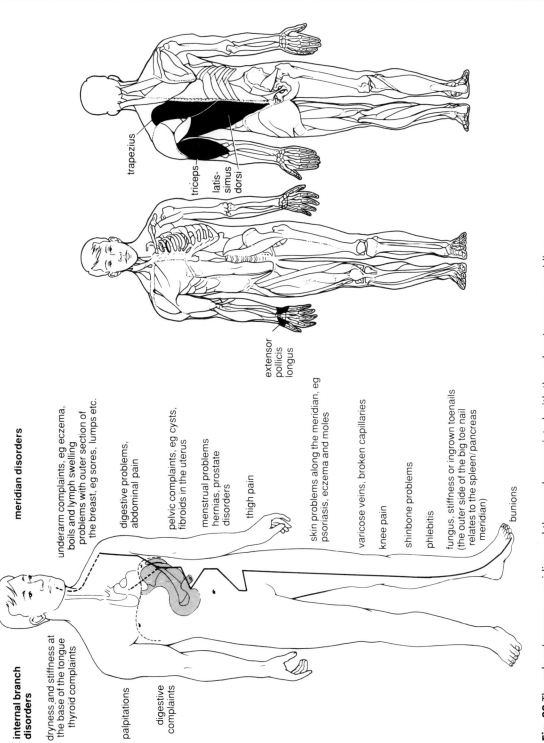

internal branch disorders

dryness and stiffness at the base of the tongue
thyroid complaints

palpitations

digestive complaints

meridian disorders

underarm complaints, eg eczema, boils and lymph swelling
problems with outer section of the breast, eg sores, lumps etc.

digestive problems, abdominal pain

pelvic complaints, eg cysts, fibroids in the uterus

menstrual problems
hernias, prostate disorders

thigh pain

skin problems along the meridian, eg psoriasis, eczema and moles

varicose veins, broken capillaries

knee pain

shinbone problems

phlebitis

fungus, stiffness or ingrown toenails (the outer side of the big toe nail relates to the spleen/pancreas meridian)

bunions

trapezius

triceps

latis-simus dorsi

extensor pollicis longus

Fig. 88 The spleen/pancreas meridian and the muscles associated with the spleen/pancreas meridian

functions of the spleen are harmonious, ch'i and blood can be abundant and digestive powers strong. If the spleen is in disharmony, the whole body or some part of it may develop deficient ch'i or deficient blood.[42] Physiologically, the pancreas has considerable control over the body's nourishment, since its secretions help digest all the main constituents of food – proteins, fats and starch.

According to the Chinese, 'The spleen governs the blood' – it helps create blood and keeps it flowing in its proper paths. It is therefore associated with blood-excreting problems and influences menstruation. The spleen also destroys spent red blood cells and forms antibodies which neutralize poisonous bacteria, influencing immunity to infection. Ch'i and blood are transported to the muscles and flesh by the spleen, therefore these too depend on the power of the spleen. Mouth and lips are closely related to the spleen. If the spleen is weak the mouth will be insensitive to taste and the lips pale.[43]

The spleen meridian has an ascending flow of energy running from the foot to the chest. It obtains its energy from the stomach meridian and passes it on to the heart meridian. The spleen/pancreas meridian starts in the centre of the back of the big toe, ascends up the leg, through the body, and ends on one side of the breast under the armpit (see diagram).

Meridian Disorders

The medial side of the big toenail relates to the spleen meridian, so fungus, stiffness or ingrown toenails here are indicative of problems of the spleen/pancreas meridian. As a reflexologist, take note of the condition of the big toe. If it points upwards, this too indicates problems with this meridian.

Bunions occur on the spleen meridian and the thyroid reflex – and if you take note of the internal branch disorders you will see that a branch of the spleen/pancreas meridian runs through the thyroid. Emotional problems are often found to be related to this meridian, for example, depression, PMT, irritability and concentration problems. Metabolic problems like goitres, fatigue, hair and nail conditions are usually related more to the stomach meridian. The spleen meridian runs along the shinbone and here you may find capillary problems; phlebitis connected to thrombosis (on the inner side of the shin); discoloration and eczema on the ankle area; knee pain on the inner side of the knee; skin problems or varicose veins along the meridian. The meridian continues up the middle of the legs so problems here could be leg and thigh pains, groin pains, hernias, pelvic complaints like cysts, fibroids in the uterus, menstrual problems, infections and prostate disorders. Pelvic problems which result in hysterectomies are often related to imbalances in the spleen/pancreas meridian.

As this meridian continues through the digestive area, problems here include abdominal pain and distension and diaphragm diseases; problems with the outer section of the breast, such as lumps, cysts, and sensitivity and swelling prior to menstruation; underarm complaints like eczema, boils and lymphatic problems.

Internal Branch Disorders

Thyroid complaints; dryness and stiffness at the base of the tongue; digestive complaints and palpitations.

Muscles Related to this Meridian

Latissimus Dorsi (*Yin*) This muscle pulls the arm down and helps keep the back straight. It is used in forceful arm movements, like swimming, rowing, bowling, golf and baseball swings. Because of its relationship with the pancreas where insulin is produced, people with diabetes, insulinaemia, hypoglycaemia or other problems of sugar metabolism will show weakness in this muscle. There will be a high shoulder on the weak side.[44]

Trapezius **(Yin)** This is one of the muscles that moves the shoulder blade. It can be involved in shoulder and arm problems.[45]

Extensor Pollicis Longus **(Yin)** If the muscles of both hands are weak and do not respond, it may indicate a fixation of the sacrum. This weakness sometimes leads to 'tennis elbow'. The wrist bones, especially the radius and ulna, are not held in a good position and strain on the elbow results. This syndrome is complicated and may require professional advice and treatment.[46]

Triceps **(Yin)** These are situated in the back of the arm and help in straightening the elbow, working opposite the biceps. They can be affected by any of the problems of sugar metabolism which affect the latissimus dorsi.[47]

HEART MERIDIAN

Yin meridian
Partner meridian Small Intestine (Yang)
Element Fire
Organ maximum energy period 11 am to 1 pm

Says the *Nei Ching*: 'The heart is like the minister of the monarch who excels through insight and understanding.'[48] And, 'The heart is the root of life and causes the versatility of the spiritual faculties. The heart influences the face and fills the pulse with blood.'[49]

The heart and small intestine meridians are coupled. The *Nei Ching* explains their relationship; 'The heart controls the blood and unites with the small intestine. If the heart becomes heated, the heat will converge in the small intestine, producing blood in the urine.'[50]

The classics also say: 'The heart rules the blood and blood vessels. Thus it regulates the blood flow, so when the heart is functioning properly, the blood flows smoothly. Therefore the heart, blood and blood vessels are united by their common activity. If the heart is strong, the body will be healthy and the emotions orderly; if it is weak, all the other meridians will be disturbed.'[51]

It is also said that the heart rules the spirit. When the heart's blood and ch'i are harmonious, spirit is nourished and the individual responds appropriately to the environment. If this is impaired, symptoms like insomnia, excessive dreaming, forgetfulness, hysteria, irrational behaviour, insanity and delirium may manifest.[52]

The heart meridian has a descending flow of energy running from the chest to the hand. It gets its ch'i from the spleen/pancreas meridian and in turn passes it on to the small intestine meridian. The heart meridian starts in the armpit and ends on the back of the little finger, towards the ring finger (see diagram).

Meridian Disorders

Pain in the armpits; swollen glands; inner arm pain and weakness; numbness, pain and stiffness of the inner aspect of the forearm; skin problems; weak wrists; stiffness, pain or numbness in the little finger; angina; nail and finger disorders like whitlows, white spots, ridges, warts or moles.

Internal Branch Disorders

Eye weakness; thirst; throat disorders; cardiac disorders; palpitations and chest pains; associated disorders of the small intestine like constipation and malabsorption, as well as diaphragm disorders.

Muscles Related to this Meridian

Subscapularis **(Yin)** This muscle cannot be seen or felt because it is behind the scapula (shoulder blade). It allows the shoulder blade to glide over the rib cage and rotates the arm backwards, drawing the arm in when it is raised above the shoulder.[53]

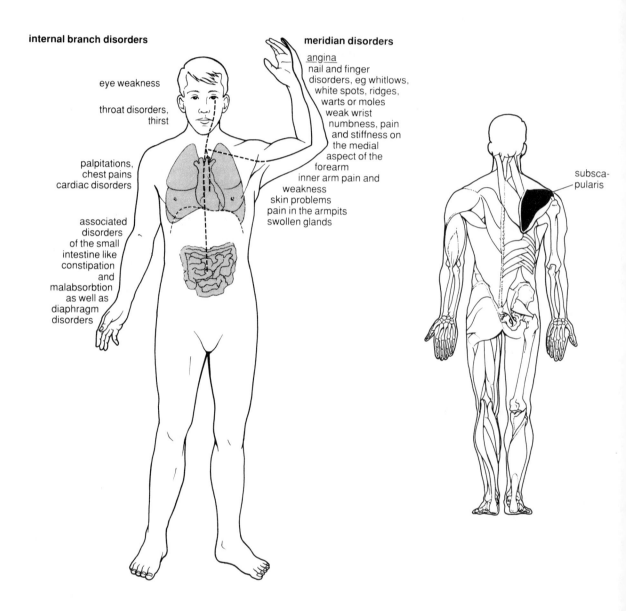

internal branch disorders

eye weakness

throat disorders, thirst

palpitations, chest pains cardiac disorders

associated disorders of the small intestine like constipation and malabsorbtion as well as diaphragm disorders

meridian disorders

<u>angina</u>
nail and finger disorders, eg whitlows, white spots, ridges, warts or moles
weak wrist
numbness, pain and stiffness on the medial aspect of the forearm
inner arm pain and weakness
skin problems
pain in the armpits
swollen glands

subsca-pularis

Fig. 89 The heart meridian and muscles associated with the heart meridian

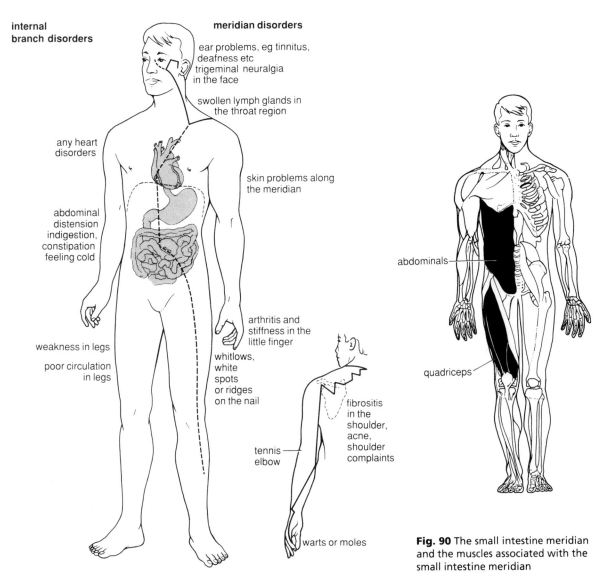

internal branch disorders

meridian disorders

ear problems, eg tinnitus, deafness etc
trigeminal neuralgia in the face

swollen lymph glands in the throat region

any heart disorders

skin problems along the meridian

abdominal distension indigestion, constipation feeling cold

weakness in legs

poor circulation in legs

arthritis and stiffness in the little finger

whitlows, white spots or ridges on the nail

tennis elbow

fibrositis in the shoulder, acne, shoulder complaints

warts or moles

abdominals

quadriceps

Fig. 90 The small intestine meridian and the muscles associated with the small intestine meridian

SMALL INTESTINE MERIDIAN

Yang meridian
Partner meridian Heart (Yin)
Element Fire
Organ maximum energy period 1 pm to 3 pm

'The small intestines are like officials who are entrusted with riches and they create changes of the physical substance,' says the *Nei Ching*.[54]

The small intestine rules the separation of the 'pure' and the 'impure'. It continues the process of separation and absorption begun in the stomach. The functioning of the large intestine is influenced, both directly and indirectly, by the small intestine. In addition to passing solid residue on to the large intestine, the small intestine also controls the proportion of liquid to solid matter in the faeces, reabsorbing some liquids for the body's use and passing some on to be eliminated.[55]

The sorting out process – keeping that which has nutritional value and passing on waste to where it can be removed – happens on all levels of experience, both physiological and psychological; for example, sorting out the rubbish from that which is useful in ideas, emotions and thoughts. If this sorting out function is not operating efficiently symptoms that express this confusion may arise – hearing difficulties, the inability to sort out sounds from each other, or digestion problems which are the result of poor sorting. Thus the flow relates not only to assimilation of foodstuffs but also to assimilation of experience, feelings, ideas and to spiritual nourishment.[56]

The small intestine meridian has an ascending flow of energy running from the hand to the head. It receives its ch'i from the heart meridian and passes it on to the bladder meridian. The small intestine meridian begins on the outside of the tip of the little finger, and passes upward along the posterior aspect of the forearm. It circles behind the shoulder ascends along the side of the neck to the cheek and outer corner of the eye before entering the ear.

Meridian Disorders

Arthritis and stiffness in the little finger, whitlows, white spots or ridges on the nail; skin problems along the meridian; tennis elbow; shoulder complaints; swelling, stiffness of cervical region, scapula, shoulders and lateral aspect of arm; fibrositis in the shoulder blade; acne; swollen lymph glands in the throat; trigeminal neuralgia in the face; ear problems like tinnitus, deafness and any other problems related to the ears.

Internal Branch Disorders

Any heart disorders; abdominal distension;

headaches; poor circulation in legs; indigestion; constipation; feeling cold; weakness in legs.

Muscles Related to this Meridian

Quadriceps (Yang) These straighten the knee and flex the thigh. Weakness will be evident when there is difficulty climbing stairs, getting up and down from a seated position, picking the knee up, pain in the kneecap and other knee problems.[57]

Abdominals (Yang) These muscles help keep the organs in place and bend the torso forwards and sideways. The rectus abdominis goes up and down the centre of the torso; the transverse abdominis is underneath going crosswise. They are associated with the duodenum, the first third of the small intestine, and are commonly involved in indigestion, 'stomach aches' and breathing difficulties. Weakness of these muscles can result in a feeling of weakness or pain in the lower back. If weakness is only on one side, there may be some restriction of shoulder movement on the opposite side.[58]

BLADDER MERIDIAN

Yang Meridian
Partner meridian Kidney (Yin)
Element Water
Organ maximum energy period 3 pm to 5 pm

'The groins and the bladder are like the magistrates of a region, they store the overflow and the fluid secretions which serve to regulate vaporisation,' says the *Nei Ching*.[59]

The partnership of the kidney and bladder meridians is one of the most obvious. The function of the bladder is to receive and excrete urine produced in the kidneys from the final portion of turbid fluids transmitted from the lungs, small intestine and large intestine. It is therefore in charge of maintaining normal fluid levels in the body. It is not merely an excretory

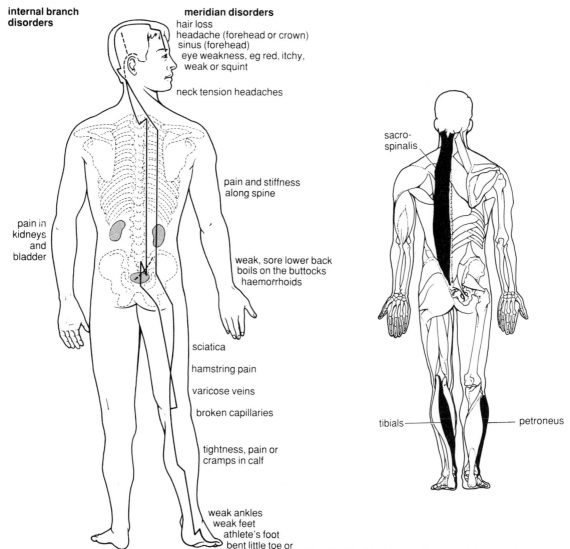

internal branch disorders

meridian disorders
hair loss
headache (forehead or crown)
sinus (forehead)
eye weakness, eg red, itchy,
  weak or squint

neck tension headaches

pain and stiffness
along spine

pain in
kidneys
and
bladder

weak, sore lower back
boils on the buttocks
haemorrhoids

sciatica

hamstring pain

varicose veins

broken capillaries

tightness, pain or
cramps in calf

weak ankles
weak feet
athlete's foot
bent little toe or
pigeon toes

sacro-
spinalis

tibials

petroneus

Fig. 91 The bladder meridian and the muscles associated with the bladder meridian

organ but is coupled with the function of the kidneys in helping to store the Jing or vital essence (refer to kidney meridian). The bladder is essential to life. If it is not functioning properly, the rest of the system is stressed and poisoned.[60]

The bladder meridian has a pronounced effect on the spinal cord and nerves, and is most effective in releasing tension along its path.

This meridian has a descending flow of energy running from the head to the foot. It receives its energy from the small intestine and passes it on to the kidney meridian. It is the longest meridian line in the body.

The bladder meridian starts at the inner corner of the eye, continues over the crown of the head, down the back and legs, and ends on the outer edge of the back of the little toe (see diagram).

Meridian Disorders

Eye weaknesses, for example red, itchy, weak or squint eyes; headaches in the crown of the head, forehead, crossing over the head, and neck tension headaches; forehead sinus; hair loss; pain and stiffness along the spine; skin problems along the meridian; weak, sore lower back; haemorrhoids; boils on the buttocks; hamstring pains. On the backs of the legs one may find sciatica; varicose veins; tightness and pain or cramps in the calf or outer ankle; weak ankles; weak feet; athlete's foot; bent little toes or pigeon toes. A minor physical defect often found in young children is a tendency to walk with their feet turned inwards. This may be combined with a tendency to bedwetting and weak eyes – all problems along the bladder meridian. If the kidney/bladder reflexes are strengthened these problems will be rectified. My younger son was born with pigeon toes and a weak bladder. For some time he had a problem with bedwetting, which we corrected with reflexology treatments. However, if he overloads his kidney/bladder system, before long his feet turn inwards again and we know it is time for more treatment.

Take note of the organs through which the bladder meridian passes, for example, the stomach and the liver. It can therefore have a marked effect on the digestive system. It also passes through the lungs and the pelvic region. The meridian runs through the lumbar vertebrae, and therefore has an indirect effect on the ovaries, testes, uterus and prostate, as the nerves from lumbar vertebrae 3 and 4 relate to these organs.

Note, too, that the stomach meridian also starts at the eye. If the bladder is overloaded, the eyes often become watery, which can also be due to excess stomach acidity. The eyes will then attempt to expel some of the excess acidity which will cause red, sensitive or sore eyes. Also remember that the stomach meridian runs through the liver so spots before the eyes and liver spots may also be due to stomach problems.

Internal Branch Disorders

Pain in the kidneys and bladder.

Muscles Related to this Meridian

Peroneus (Yang) This is the lower leg muscle which flexes the side of the foot upward and out. Weakness will cause the foot to turn in, especially in children, and can also be associated with ankle and foot problems.[61]

Sacrospinalis (Yang) This is a group of several separate muscles along the backbone. It can be the cause of nineteen different areas of pain and malfunction in the spine and is associated with problems of arthritis, rheumatism, bursitis, shoulder and elbow problems and even snapping fingers. Weakness on one side will cause a bending of the spine which can become a serious problem if neglected. Both sides weak will create the posture seen on many skinny people; the abdominal muscles contracted, the head and hips forward and the spine pushed back. This muscle is closely associated with bladder problems and may also be affected by emotional strain.[62]

Tibialis Anterior (Yang) This muscle flexes the foot in and upwards and is often found weak on both sides. Weakness can be associated with rectal fissures, and urethra and bladder problems.[64]

KIDNEY MERIDIAN

Yin Meridian
Partner Meridian Bladder (Yang)
Element Water
Organ maximum energy period 5 pm to 7 pm

'The kidneys are like officials who do energetic work and they excel through their ability,' says

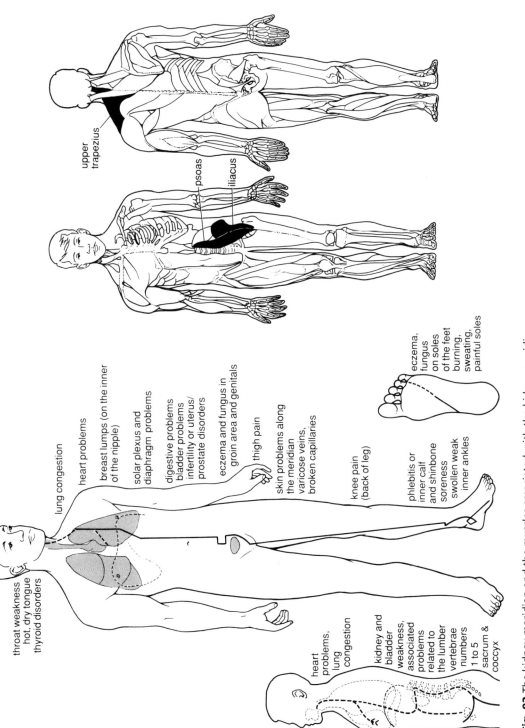

internal branch disorders

meridian disorders

throat weakness
hot, dry tongue
thyroid disorders

lung congestion

heart problems

breast lumps (on the inner
of the nipple)

solar plexus and
diaphragm problems

digestive problems
bladder problems
infertility or uterus/
prostate disorders

eczema and fungus in
groin area and genitals

thigh pain

skin problems along
the meridian
varicose veins,
broken capillaries

knee pain
(back of leg)

phlebitis or
inner calf
and shinbone
soreness
swollen weak
inner ankles

eczema,
fungus
on soles
of the feet
burning,
sweating,
painful soles

heart
problems,
lung
congestion

kidney and
bladder
weakness,
associated
problems
related to
the lumber
vertebrae
numbers
1 to 5
sacrum &
coccyx

upper
trapezius

psoas

iliacus

Fig. 92 The kidney meridian and the muscles associated with the kidney meridian

the *Nei Ching*.[64] And: 'The kidneys call to life that which is dormant and sealed up; they are the natural organ for storing away, and they are the place where the secretions are lodged. The kidneys influence the hair on the head and have an effect upon the bones.[65]

The kidneys store the jing and rule birth, development and maturation. Jing is the substance – a vital essence – which is the source of life and individual development. It has the potential for development into yin and yang and therefore produces life. The body and all the organs need jing to survive, and because the kidneys store jing, they bestow this potential for life activity. They therefore have a special relationship with the other organs because the yin and yang, or life activity, of each organ ultimately depends on the yin and yang of the kidneys. Jing is the source of reproduction, development and maturation, so all these processes are governed by the kidneys. Reproductive energy is produced manifesting as sperm and ova.[66]

The kidneys regulate the amount of water in the body. fluid is essential to life as it bathes the entire cellular system. The flow of fluid enables waste material to be collected and excreted in the form of urine. Enormous amounts of blood flow through the kidneys to be purified and broken down into nutritional components for the body.[67]

The kidneys rule the bones and produce marrow. As the teeth are related to bone, they too are ruled by the kidneys. There is also a close relationship between the kidneys and the ears, and normal breathing also requires assistance from the kidneys. They also influence the adrenal glands and parathyroids as well as having a close connection with the spinal column, as the kidney meridian ascends the spine to the skull.[68]

The kidney meridian has an ascending flow of energy running from the foot to the chest. It receives ch'i from the bladder and passes it on to the pericardium meridian.

The kidney meridian starts on the sole of the foot and ascends up the back of the leg. It emerges around the front of the lower thigh and ascends straight up the body to the breast bone (see diagram).

Meridian Disorders

Burning, painful soles of the feet; eczema and fungus on the soles of the feet; weak, swollen inner ankles; shinbone sores; phlebitis on inner calves; knee pain (back of leg); thigh pain; varicose veins, broken capillaries, skin problems along the meridian; eczema and fungus in groin area and genitals; sexual problems like infertility or uterus/prostate disorders; bladder weakness; digestive problems in the small intestine or colon; solar plexus and diaphragm problems; breast problems; lumps in the breast on the inner sides of the nipple; hip problems; tightness in the chest area; asthma; lung congestion.

Internal Branch Disorders

Kidney and bladder weakness; pains in the spine – associated problems related to the lumbar vertebrae numbers 1 to 5; pain; lung congestion; throat weakness, coughs; hot dry tongue, thyroid disorders.

Muscles Related to this Meridian

Psoas (Yin) This is part of the spine-flexing group and helps keep the lumbar curve in the spine. With weakness on both sides there will be a tendency for the lower back to flatten. Weakness on one side will cause the foot to turn in or make the hip low. Standing or walking with the ankles turned in will put a strain on the psoas and can cause recurring weakness if the foot problem is not corrected. Nagging low back pain, kidney disturbances and foot problems can be associated with psoas weakness.[69]

Upper Trapezius (Yin) This muscle tilts the head back and pulls the shoulder blade up. This will weaken with any problems associated with the ears and eyes.[70]

Iliacus (Yin) This muscle, if weak, may indicate a problem with the ileo-caecal valve, the muscular valve between the small and large intestines. If the muscles are weak an extensive set of symptoms may develop including nausea, sudden low back pain, shoulder pain, headache, sudden thirst, dark circles under the eyes and pallor.[71]

PERICARDIUM/CIRCULATION MERIDIAN

Yin meridian
Partner meridian Triple burner (Yang)
Element Fire
Organ maximum energy period 7 pm to 9 pm

It is said that diseases of the heart are borne by the pericardium. The pericardium is the outer protective shield of the heart – a loose fibrous sac which encloses a slippery lubricated membrane to prevent friction as the heart beats. Its role is to defend the heart from stress, shocks and other harmful influences. The West does not recognize this particular system as an organ and technically it is not. But the Chinese appreciated that an organ does not have to be in one piece to be effective, so they considered the whole vascular system to be an organ within itself. It covers the arteries, veins and capillaries which deal with the circulation of fluid in the body. The pericardium meridian is also known as the heart constrictor, heart circulation or circulation meridian. The pericardium and triple burner are partner meridians. Both have numerous names and protective functions, and neither is an organ in the strict technical sense of the word. If the triple burner is imbalanced, the organs are deprived of proper nourishment and revolt against the heart; if the pericardium is weak, the heart will be attacked and the nourishing activities of the triple burner will be less effective.[72]

The pericardium meridian has a descending flow of energy running from the chest to the hand. It obtains its ch'i from the kidney meridian, and passes it on to the triple burner meridian. The meridian starts next to the nipple and descends down the arm ending on the back of the middle finger, towards the ring finger (see diagram).

Meridian Disorders

Swollen, painful armpits; eczema or skin problems in the elbow crease; skin problems along the arm on the medial aspect; carpal tunnel syndrome; hot palms; arthritis/eczema in the middle finger; any nail disorders of the middle finger.

Internal Branch Disorders

Hot flushes and rapid heart beat; heart pain; diaphragm constriction; endocrine-related problems.

Muscles Related to this Meridian

Gluteus Minimus (Yin) This is used to pull the leg out sideways and rotate it inwards. If there is weakness in this muscle, the hip and shoulder may be high, and there is also a tendency towards bowed legs or a peculiar limp.[73]

Adductors (Yin) These hold the thigh in and rotate it inward. Weakness can make the pelvis tilt down, will sometimes complicate stiff shoulders and can even cause elbow pain. Problems with the reproductive organs, especially changes in hormone function or menopause, can affect the adductors.[74]

Piriformis (Yin) This hip muscle is very important in posture, especially the position of the sacrum. It is the uppermost of the hip rotators. In a seated position it allows the leg to move outward. Weakness on one side can cause the sacrum to twist, making the ankle on that side turn in, the knees 'knock', and the opposite

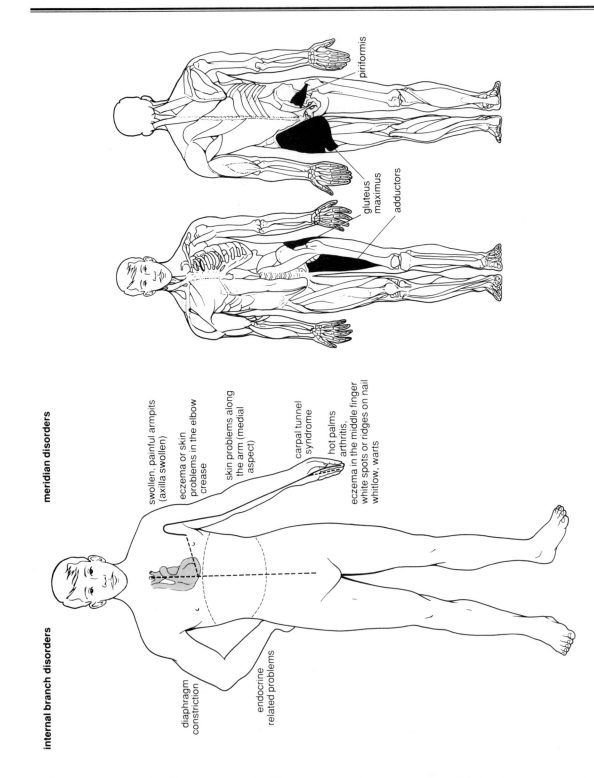

meridian disorders

piriformis

gluteus maximus

adductors

swollen, painful armpits (axilla swollen)

eczema or skin problems in the elbow crease

skin problems along the arm (medial aspect)

carpal tunnel syndrome

hot palms arthritis, eczema in the middle finger white spots or ridges on nail whitlow, warts

internal branch disorders

diaphragm constriction

endocrine related problems

Fig. 93 The pericardium meridian and the muscles associated with the pericardium meridian

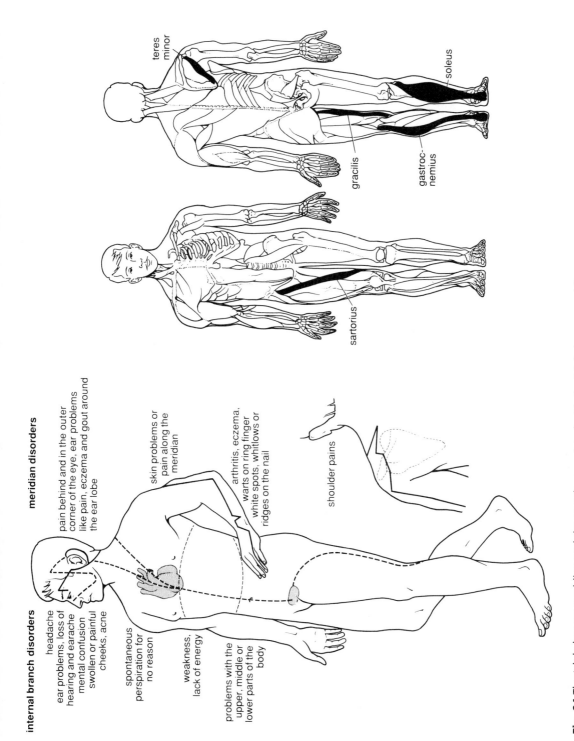

internal branch disorders

headache
ear problems. loss of
hearing and earache
mental confusion
swollen or painful
cheeks, acne

spontaneous
perspiration for
no reason

weakness,
lack of energy

problems with the
upper, middle or
lower parts of the
body

meridian disorders

pain behind and in the outer
corner of the eye, ear problems
like pain, eczema and gout around
the ear lobe

skin problems or
pain along the
meridian

arthritis, eczema,
warts on ring finger
white spots, whitlows or
ridges on the nail

shoulder pains

teres
minor

soleus

gracilis

gastroc-
nemius

sartorius

Fig. 94 The triple burner meridian and the muscles associated with the triple burner meridian

foot turn out. It is located right next to the sciatic nerve (the longest, largest nerve in the body), and problems with this muscle can often affect the sciatic nerve. There may be pain down the leg, numbness and tingling of the legs, burning urine and other bladder problems.[75]

Gluteus Maximus (Yin) This is one of the largest and strongest muscles in the body. It acts as a stabilizer of the lower back and extends the thigh. Weakness of one side will twist the pelvis or make the crease of the buttocks go off to one side. With both sides weak, walking is difficult.[76]

TRIPLE BURNER MERIDIAN

Yang meridian
Partner Meridian Pericardium (Yin)
Element Fire
Organ maximum energy period 9 pm to 11 pm

Says the **Nei Ching**: 'The three burning spaces are like the officials who plan the construction of ditches and sluices and they create waterways.'[77]

The triple burner is not exactly an organ, but a relationship between various organs. The Chinese saw it as being composed of three sections which control the chemical activity within the body, regulate and adjust body temperature changes, and transfer ch'i from one area to another. The three 'heaters', 'warmers' or 'burners' correspond to three divisions of the body: the upper burner to the thoracic cavity including the heart and lungs; the middle burner to the upper abdominal cavity including the spleen/pancreas and the stomach; and the lower burner to the lower abdominal cavity which encompasses the liver and kidneys, intestines and bladder.[78]

This meridian governs activities involving all the organs and unites the respiratory, digestive and excretory systems. It may be related to the hypothalamus, the link between the nervous

system and endocrine glands. Its functions include:

1. regulation of the autonomic nervous system, thus of the heart and abdominal organs especially in their response to emotion;
2. control of the pituitary (which regulates the output of all the endocrine glands);
3. regulation of body temperature, appetite and thirst;
4. control of emotions and moods, influencing social relations.[79]

The triple burner meridian has an ascending flow of energy running from the hand to the head. It receives its ch'i from the pericardium meridian and passes it on to the gall bladder meridian. The meridian starts on the back of the ring finger, ascends up the arm and ends at the top of the outer corner of the eye (see diagram).

Meridian Disorders

Disorders of the ring finger like arthritis and nail problems; eczema on this finger and along the meridian; stiffness and pain along the arm and wrist; shoulder pains; ear problems such as pain, eczema and gout around the ear lobe; pain behind and in the outer corner of the eye.

Internal Branch Disorders

Ear problems – loss of hearing and earache; spontaneous perspiration for no reason; mental confusion; weakness; lack of energy; swollen or painful cheeks; acne; problems with the upper, middle or lower portions of the body.

Muscles Related to this Meridian

Teres Minor (Yang) This is the shoulder muscle which rotates the arm and can be involved in wrist and elbow problems. With weakness on one side, the hands will be turned differently when the arms hang down to the side.[80]

Sartorius (Yang) This thigh muscle helps to

flex the thigh and rotate it outwards. It is the longest muscle in the body. Weakness will cause the pelvis to twist and it can also be the cause of knee pain or knock knees because of the resulting instability of the knee joint. Adrenal problems can affect this muscle.[81]

Gracilis (Yang) This thigh muscle pulls the leg inwards. When lying down it is the first muscle used when bending the knee. Weakness makes it difficult to bend the knee without flexing the hip. Adrenal problems can be related to this muscle.[82]

Soleus (Yang) This is the calf muscle which flexes the foot and the lower part of the leg, steadying the foot. Weakness may cause a forward lean of the body or bending of the knees. Adrenal problems can affect this muscle.[83]

Gastrocnemius (Yang) This calf muscle works with the soleus in flexing the foot and lower part of the leg. Weakness can cause hyperextension of the knee (knee pushed too far back), inability to rise up on the toes, or difficulty bending the knee.[84]

GALL BLADDER MERIDIAN

Yang meridian
Partner meridian Liver (Yin)
Element Wood
Organ maximum energy period 11 pm to 1 am

'The gall bladder occupies the position of an important and upright official who excels through his decision and judgement,' says the *Nei Ching*.[85]

The attitudes of all the other organs originate in the energy of the gall bladder, according to the ancients. The gall bladder is different from all the other organs in that they transport 'impure' or foreign matter – food, liquid and the waste products thereof. Only the gall bladder transports 'pure' liquids exclusively.[86]

The gall bladder stores and secretes bile – a bitter yellow fluid continuously produced by the liver – and sends this bile down into the intestine where it aids the digestive process. Any disruptions of the liver will affect the gall bladder's bile secretion and disharmonies of the gall bladder will affect the liver.

This meridian is one of the most well travelled, traversing almost the entire body except the arms. It zig-zags throughout the head in a pattern which, in times of stress and tension, becomes like a vice and is therefore important in cases of headaches, neck tension and 'uptightness'.[87]

The *Nei Ching* says the gall bladder rules decisions, so angry behaviour and rash decisions may indicate an excess of gall bladder ch'i, while indecision and timidity may be signs of gall bladder disharmony and weakness.[88]

The gall bladder meridian has a descending flow of energy running from the head to the foot. It receives its ch'i from the triple burner meridian and passes it on to the liver meridian.

The gall bladder meridian starts at the outer corner of the eye, traverses the temple and descends to the shoulder. It continues laterally down the body and leg to end on the back of the fourth toe, towards the little toe (see diagram).

Meridian Disorders

Shooting pains lateral to the eye; eye weakness; temple headaches/migraines; neck tension; jaw pain; ear weakness; pain and stiffness in the trapezius; shoulder pain from, for example, a frozen shoulder; pain and tightness in the ribs; asthma; shingles; arthritis/pain in the hip – shooting pains from front to back or vice versa; skin problems along the meridian; knee complaints on the lateral side of the knee; puffiness on the hip reflex of the foot; corns, athlete's foot, fungus, hammertoe or any other disorders on the fourth toe.

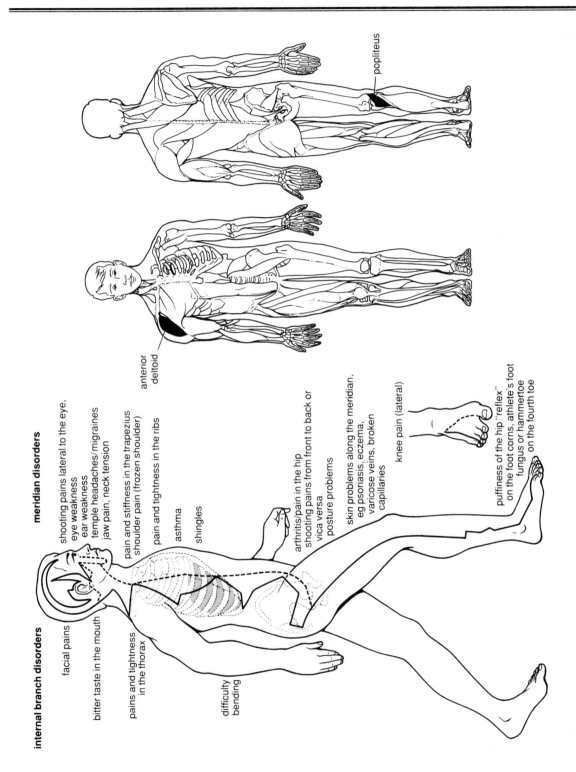

popliteus

anterior
deltoid

meridian disorders

shooting pains lateral to the eye,
eye weakness
ear weakness
temple headaches/migraines
jaw pain, neck tension

pain and stiffness in the trapezius
shoulder pain (frozen shoulder)

pain and tightness in the ribs

asthma

shingles

arthritis/pain in the hip
shooting pains from front to back or
vica versa
posture problems

skin problems along the meridian,
eg psoriasis, eczema,
varicose veins, broken
capillaries

knee pain (lateral)

puffiness of the hip "reflex"
on the foot corns, athlete's foot
fungus or hammertoe
on the fourth toe

internal branch disorders

facial pains

bitter taste in the mouth

pains and tightness
in the thorax

difficulty
bending

Fig. 95 The gall bladder meridian and the muscles associated with the gall bladder meridian

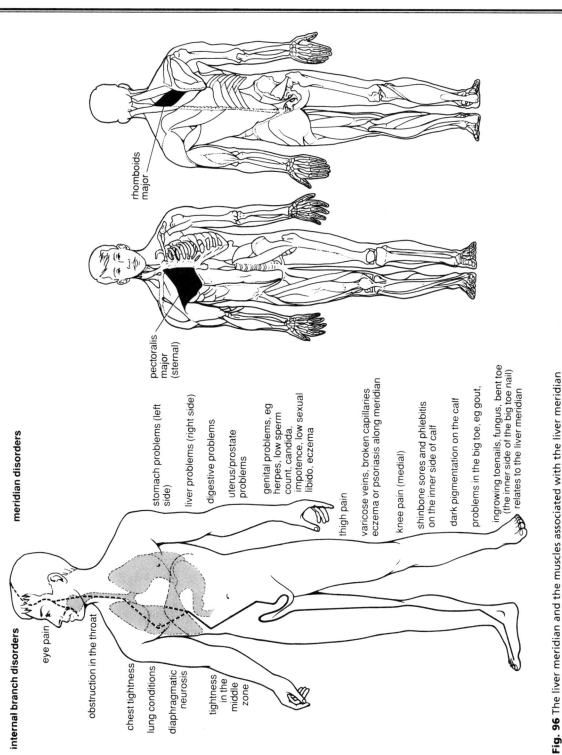

rhomboids major

pectoralis major (sternal)

internal branch disorders

meridian disorders

eye pain

obstruction in the throat

chest tightness

lung conditions

diaphragmatic neurosis

tightness in the middle zone

stomach problems (left side)

liver problems (right side)

digestive problems

uterus/prostate problems

genital problems, eg herpes, low sperm count, candida, impotence, low sexual libido, eczema

thigh pain

varicose veins, broken capillaries eczema or psoriasis along meridian

knee pain (medial)

shinbone sores and phlebitis on the inner side of calf

dark pigmentation on the calf

problems in the big toe, eg gout,

ingrowing toenails, fungus, bent toe (the inner side of the big toe nail) relates to the liver meridian

Fig. 96 The liver meridian and the muscles associated with the liver meridian

Internal Branch Disorders

Bitter taste in the mouth; facial pains; pains and tightness in the thorax; difficulty bending.

Muscles Related to the Meridian

Anterior Deltoid (Yang) This muscle is used along with the coracobrachialis in flexing the shoulder with the elbow bent, as in combing the hair. It is not usually found to be weak, but could be related to many headache cases which are caused by toxicity from bad diet.[89]

Popliteus (Yang) This muscle turns the lower leg in. Problems here could be hyperextension of the knee (knee pushed too far back), and bending the knee may become difficult or painful.[90]

LIVER MERIDIAN

Yin Meridian
Partner meridian Gall Bladder (Yang)
Element Wood
Organ maximum energy period 1 am to 3 am

'The liver has the functions of a military leader who excels in his strategic planning,' says the *Nei Ching*.[91] And: 'The liver causes utmost weariness and is the dwelling place of the soul, or spiritual part of man that ascends to heaven. The liver influences the nails and is effective upon the muscles; it brings forth animal desires and vigour.'[92]

According to the *Nei Ching*, the liver rules 'flowing' and 'spreading'. The liver or liver ch'i is responsible for smooth movement of bodily substances and for regularity of body activities. It moves ch'i and blood in all directions, sending them to every part of the body, and maintains evenness and harmony of movement throughout the body. All activity that depends on ch'i depends also on the liver. Any impairment of liver function can influence the circulation of ch'i and blood.[93]

The liver controls bile secretions and is involved in storage and regulation of blood. It is the primary centre of metabolism – it synthesizes proteins, neutralizes poisons and regulates blood sugar levels; stores glycogen (starch), and changes it back to glucose (sugar) when needed for energy. Since the brain does not store any glucose, the liver's steady supply is crucial to life, and this is why the Chinese saw the liver as vital to conscious and unconscious thought, and responsible for creating a relaxed internal environment.[94]

Emotional disruptions will affect the functions of the liver, which will in turn affect the emotional state. Anger, depression and emotional frustrations are associated with the liver. Balance in this meridian will produce a sense of well-being and reasonable temperament.[95] In China, it is said that the 'liver governs the eyes' and many eye complaints can be related to the liver. The tendons are also related to the liver.

The liver meridian has an ascending flow of energy running from the foot to the chest. It receives ch'i from the gall bladder meridian and passes it on to the lung meridian.

The liver meridian starts on the back of the big toe and ascends medially up the leg to the genital region. From there it continues upwards to just below the nipple on the lower part of the breast bone (see diagram).

Meridian Disorders

Symptoms on the big toe like gout, ingrown toenails, fungus of the toenail, bent toe; shin-bone sores and phlebitis on the inner side of the calf; dark pigmentation on the calf; pain on the medial side of the knee; thigh pain; eczema or psoriasis along the thighs or meridian; varicose veins; eczema, fungus and pains in the groin area; genital problems like herpes, low sperm count, impotence, low sexual libido, candida, uterus and prostate problems; digestive problems; liver problems on the right side; stomach and spleen/

pancreas problems on the left side; pains and tightness in the ribs. When the elderly have circulation problems, brown patches are often seen along the liver meridian. On alcoholics I have seen sores which will not heal along the liver meridian.

Internal Branch Disorders

Eye pain; obstructions in the throat; chest tightness; lung conditions; tightness in the middle zone; diaphragm disorders.

Muscles Related to this Meridian

Pectoralis Major (*Sternal*) (*Yin*) This is responsible for moving the arm in, turning and drawing it forward.[96]

Rhomboids (*Yin*) These muscles in the back of the shoulders pull the shoulder blades together and upwards. They are used with the levator scapulae and are rarely found to be weak. [97]

SPECIAL MERIDIANS

Two special meridians, referred to as 'vessels', the governing vessel and conception vessel, are considered major meridians. This is because they have independent points – points that are not on any of the twelve regular meridians.[98] These two vessels run along the midline of the body – front and back – to form what seems to be the central body circuit. They are not part of the general circulatory system but are related to it as a secondary channel.[99]

GOVERNING VESSEL

A yang meridian, this acts mainly on the yang energy, having a governing effect on all the other yang meridians and organs – small intestine, triple burner, stomach, large intestine, bladder and gall bladder. The yang organ functions are

primarily active and relate to the breaking down of food and fluids and the absorption of nutrients from them, the circulation of the derived 'nourishing energies' around the body, and the secretion of unused materials.[100] The three yang meridians found in the feet are the largest, covering a large portion of the body. When the body is bent forward, the meridians have an 'outside' path, which is characteristic of yang meridians. The energy flow is ascendent running from the coccyx to the upper gum.

The governing vessel begins in the pelvic cavity, and ascends along the middle of the spinal column to penetrate the brain. The main branch continues over the top of the head, descends across the forehead and nose to end inside the upper gum. An internal branch starts in the pelvic cavity, ascends through the tip of the coccyx to reach the kidneys in the lumbar region.[101]

Right on the top of the head is a special connecting point for all yang meridians. According to Chinese philosophy it is a point of contact of the heavenly yang. The name of the point is 'Baihui' which means 'meeting point for 100 points'. This point governs all other points and meridians in the body.[102]

Muscles related to this meridian

Teres major This muscle in the back of the shoulder draws the arm in and keeps it turned out.[103]

CONCEPTION VESSEL

This is a yin vessel which has a governing effect on all the other yin meridians. Via its connection with the yin meridians from the foot, it has a special effect on the lowest of the three burners, and thereby on the ability to conceive. The tin meridians and organ functions – heart, pericardium, spleen/pancreas, lungs, kidneys

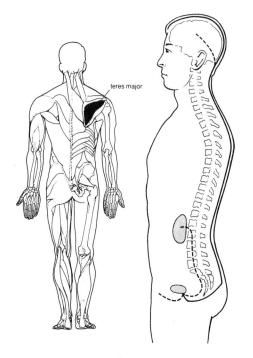

Fig. 97 The governing vessel and associated muscles

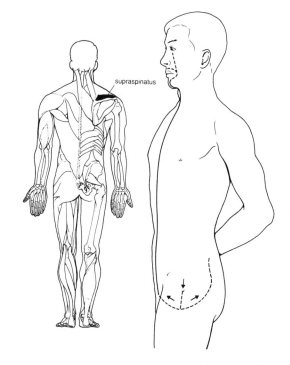

Fig. 98 The conception vessel and associated muscles

and liver – are related to the storing of vital essence. They have to do with the generation, regulation, transformation and storage of energy, blood, fluids, and spirit (shen). Yin functions are conceived of as deeper and more essential for vital functioning than the yang functions.[104] The energy flow is ascendent, running from the perineum to the chin.

The conception vessel starts from the pelvic cavity and runs forward across the pubic region. It ascends along the midline of the abdomen, through the chest. It then passes up the throat to the lower jaw. An internal branch encircles the lips and branches up to the eyes.[105]

The special connecting point for all yin meridians is situated at the base of the sternum where, according to the *Nei Ching*, all the energies are collected. This meridian penetrates the solar plexus, and could thus have some relationship to the symbolism described by Omraam Mikhaël Aïvanhov in Section 1: Chapter 2.

Muscles related to this meridian

Supraspinatus This muscle helps in moving the arm away from the body and in holding the arm into the shoulder socket, so it can be involved in shoulder problems.[106]

CHAPTER THREE

Meridian Case Histories

A reflexologist is a therapist who uses the science of stimulating reflexes in the feet to encourage the body to heal itself. In most countries, reflexologists are not allowed to diagnose specific conditions. As a teacher and practitioner, I have found it imperative that the client understands the nature of their complaints, so they are more inclined to co-operate with any suggested advice. In order to do this, a practitioner requires a detailed case history of all symptoms and problems. With a clear idea of the symptoms, the practitioner can refer and relate the complaints to the meridians and thereby ascertain which organs are out of balance. So, instead of diagnosing a medical condition according to the symptoms, one must understand these in accordance with the Chinese meridian system to equate them with congestion in energy flow.

Careful study of the paths of the twelve meridians will show that the stomach meridian penetrates all the major organs in the body, as well as passing through the reflexes of all the major organs on the feet. Therefore, this is the dominant meridian, and often the root cause of congestions. Problems will obviously affect the partner meridian, the spleen/pancreas, as well as the other meridians. The root congestion will manifest as different symptoms in different people, but 90 per cent of the time, the stomach and its meridian are involved.

In case histories where problems are found in the arms and hands, these are related to the lung, large intestine, pericardium, triple burner, small intestine and heart meridians. None of these meridians penetrates any of the major organs of the body but a problem with an organ can cause a blockage in the ch'i in the arms and hands, resulting in uncomfortable symptoms – for example, pains in the thumbs mentioned in the first meridian case history below.

Therefore, it is of vital importance to carry out a complete reflexology treatment, no matter what the symptoms, rather than work on the isolated reflexes one may think are congested. The actual organs may not phsyically exhibit any specific weakness, but problems may be expressed in congestions of ch'i at any point along a meridian. As an example, refer to the case histories related to the large intestine meridian; the main symptoms were problems on the arms and face, yet the condition arose from a large intestine imbalance. The same applies to all the other case histories mentioned which describe meridians in the arms – for example, the heart, small intestine, pericardium and triple burner meridians.

The kidney and bladder meridians are partner meridians, and the main symptoms which illustrate imbalance in these organs are headaches, weak eyes, neck tension and back problems, and to some degree sciatica and leg problems. Disease in the liver and gall bladder, also partner meridians, often manifests as migraines, gout, nausea, gallstones, frozen shoulder, hip and lateral leg complaints, and sexual problems.

Each case history has been described so that you can relate the most obvious symptoms to blockages along specific meridians, but, as mentioned earlier, one will usually find numerous symptoms and operations directly related to the stomach, spleen/pancreas and their meridians. Therefore, a change in diet will always have positive results.

The following case histories have all been effectively treated with the reflexology techniques described in this book. To more fully understand symptoms along the meridians and therefore the case histories, refer to the meridian illustrations.

LUNG MERIDIAN

Female: Age – 30s

The main reason the client sought treatment was severe pain in the 'nerve' in both thumbs.

Other symptoms: Feels a 'total mess' – allergies, skin problems, rashes on her face and scalp, frequent blocked nose, headaches (forehead and neck). Wine makes her nauseous. Discontinued contraceptive pills three to four months previously. Periods are now regular, but had been heavy and painful. Suffers slight constipation.

On studying the case history, one notices obvious symptoms related to the stomach, spleen/pancreas and their meridians, such as allergies, rashes on the face, heavy painful periods and slight constipation. But the reason she sought treatment was the pain in her thumbs,

which indicates a blockage in the ch'i energy of the lung meridian.

Female: Age – 35

Symptoms: Pins and needles in upper foot (lung reflex area), pins and needles in the fingers, specifically the index finger and thumb. Muscular problems; chest problems; fluid on the lungs; constipation or diarrhoea; pain along the stomach meridian on the left side from the ovary upwards; hiatus hernia.

Previous Operations: Hysterectomy; bladder repair; appendectomy.

Pins and needles in the fingers indicate congestions relating to the large intestine (index finger) and the lungs (thumb). Problems on the lung reflex on the feet confirm the body warning of chest weakness. This is evident in her chest problems. Constipation/diarrhoea confirm the problems in the large intestine relating to the index finger. The appendix and ovaries are situated on the stomach meridian, and problems here indicate an imbalance in the stomach. The hysterectomy can also be seen as an imbalance in the spleen/pancreas meridian, the stomach's partner meridian. There is also a strong possibility that the stomach is the root cause of all the problems, as the stomach meridian also runs through the large intestine and lung.

Reflexology techniques and the lung meridian

Many reflexology students have trouble executing the thumb techniques due to painful thumbs. Some even consider giving up reflexology because of the pain. They often think they're not applying the technique correctly. However, on checking their technique, I have found nothing wrong but question them about possible lung problems. Some have had symptoms indicating an imbalance in the lung meridian – for example, shortness of breath, bronchial problems and the like. If painful thumbs are a problem for you, look into the state of balance in the lungs and correct that before considering giving up reflexology.

LARGE INTESTINE MERIDIAN

Female: Age – 38

Symptoms: As a teenager she had a wart on her right index finger. She suffered from cold sores on the lips and inside the nose four times a year, for which treatment was required. Constipation; nervous stomach which would progress into painful colic if left unattendend. Colds invariably developed into chest problems and occasionally pneumonia. As soon as she disrupts her diet, she develops fever, blisters on her lips and sores in her nose, and the wart scar becomes sore and itchy. These are all symptoms found along the large intestine meridian – and when the sores erupt, they are warning signals of overloading this organ.

As mentioned in the introduction to this chapter, none of the meridians in the arms penetrates the major organs. But organs related to the meridians in the arms – in this case, the large intestine – are penetrated by the stomach and other meridians, and the cause will therefore usually be found in one or more of the major organs and their meridians.

Female: Age – mid 50s

Symptoms: Pain in upper right arm from forearm to index finger. The arm sometimes goes into spasm. This condition has existed for three years. Neck tension; constipation (takes laxatives regularly); slow digestion; had a hiatus hernia; meningitis as a child; one short leg; backache.

Previous Operations: Appendectomy; and an operation for endometriosis.

As in the previous case, the main problems were with her arms, which indicates congestions along the large intestine meridian. However,

one still needs to study and stimulate all the other organs and their meridians.

STOMACH MERIDIAN

Female: Age – 35

Symptoms: The client sought help for a constant blocked nose which was causing severe sinus problems. She had gained weight following a hysterectomy, and was taking oestrogen and primrin for ovarian problems. She had a weak bladder and suffered cramps in her calf muscles at night. Before having a hysterectomy, she had ovarian pains, irregular periods and sore breasts around the outer area (pancreas meridian). The operation eliminated these problems. This also occurs when one takes contraceptive pills. The symptoms of imbalance are suppressed, but the cause is not dealt with so the congestion still exists.

Previous Operations: Hiatus hernia; hysterectomy.

The congestions were obvious on the stomach meridian – sinus, thyroid (weight problems), ovaries – and the partner spleen/pancreas meridian – sore breasts, irregular periods and hysterectomy. Suppressed congestions will often be expressed more severely via a different outlet on the same meridian, in this case sinus and weight gain. The night cramps and weak bladder are related to the bladder meridian.

Male: Age – 60s

Symptoms: The client sought treatment for a constant dry, nervous, irritating cough which was particularly bad at night. It had persisted for years without relief. Six years previously he had contracted yellow jaundice. He also had high blood pressure.

Previous Operations: Gall bladder removed; tonsillectomy; nose operation.

His food intake was highly acidic, with very few

vegetables. This obviously had a negative effect on the stomach meridian, as all the symptoms relate to this meridian. The quality of nourishment was obviously not in harmony with the earth element. Thus the stomach – earth – exerted a negative effect on the wood element – liver/gall bladder. This can be seen from the jaundice and gall bladder removal.

Male: Age – 20s

Symptoms: The main problem for this young runner was severe knee pain on the lateral side, to the extent that his sport activities were affected. He also suffered sinus pain, tennis elbow, Gilbert's disease (a form of jaundice) and disrupted sleep which he attributed to stress.

Previous Operation: Tonsillectomy.

Knee pains can often be described as similar to the stabbing pain of a headache. Medical doctors may operate and scrape the knee, or find nothing medically wrong. However, relating this to a meridian can be more informative. This client's knee pain was situated on the stomach meridian, as were the other symptoms of sinus pain, liver problems (jaundice) and tonsil disorders. Stress can also be related to the stomach meridian as the thyroid is situated on this meridian, and stress on the stomach will disrupt the thyroid and thereby one's ability to deal with stress.

Female: Age – late 40s

Symptoms: Her menstrual cycle was creating problems. Contraceptive pills caused brown pigmentation on the face so she discontinued these and had an IUD fitted. Her menstrual cycle became irregular, heavy, long and painful, and she suffered intense PMT. Other complaints included lower back problems, hayfever, sinus, phlegm in the chest and a tendency to sore breasts.

Previous Operation: Removal of ingrown warts from throat area.

Pigmentation is often perceived as a liver complaint, even though it manifests on the stomach meridian in the face. Pigmentation on the face can indicate congestions in the ovaries as the stomach meridian penetrates the ovaries as well as the liver. This is why contraceptive pill side-effects often manifest as facial pigmentation. The menstrual cycle is also influenced by the spleen/pancreas meridian – evident in the PMT. The stomach meridian also runs through the chest and throat. An internal branch has an effect on the thyroid. The backache is on the bladder meridian, the lower region of which penetrates the lumbar vertebrae. Lumbar vertebra 3 is connected to the ovaries. Lower back pain and menstrual pain often go together.

SPLEEN/PANCREAS MERIDIAN

Female: Age – 20s

Symptoms: A severely swollen left leg brought this client to seek reflexology treatment. The leg had been swollen for three months, and doctors had diagnosed 'faulty lymph glands', for which they could offer no treatment. She also suffered frequent sore throats and nausea, felt very nervous, was on contraceptive pills and had recently lost a great deal of weight.

Previous Operation: Tonsillectomy.

The spleen is part of the lymph system and the swelling was a result of 'faulty lymphs'. The swelling had begun in the groin region of the spleen/pancreas meridian, and could be 'traced' down the leg along the meridian. Nervousness and weight loss can often be linked to a combination of thyroid and pancreas imbalance. The internal spleen/pancreas meridian runs through the throat area. Her diet was high in stimulants like tea, coffee and sugar. The tonsillectomy, nausea and sore throat can be traced to the partner meridian, the stomach.

Female: Age – 20

Symptoms: The client came for help for a spine problem she had suffered since age 14 – degeneration of the thoracic vertebrae 6 and 7. She also suffered from pain in her lower back, and painful bunions were developing. Regular menstrual cycle, but heavy and painful. She had a weak bladder; suffered headaches if she went without tea; felt ill when consuming rice or coffee; was anaemic for which she took iron supplements.

The nerve supply from thoracic vertebrae 6 and 7 is related to the stomach, pancreas and duodenum. The pancreas is concerned with digesting proteins. The problem with rice and coffee and the need for tea to calm her headaches indicate a pancreas imbalance. The heavy, painful menstrual cycle and anaemia confirm this. To strengthen the vertebrae, it is necessary to strengthen the stomach and pancreas.

HEART MERIDIAN

Female: Age – 62

Symptoms: Medical diagnosis of a weak heart – has an extra 'tick'. Pain in little finger of the left hand; aching muscles on the left side of the body, specifically the left shoulder, which can last up to three to four weeks; middle ear imbalance. Other symptoms included constipation, nausea which sometimes persists for up to four weeks; instant migraines after eating chocolate or cheese; high blood pressure; problems with menstrual cycle – still has periods despite her age; had cramps which stopped when she started taking contraceptive pills.

Previous Operations: Appendectomy; bunion removal twenty years before; three cysts removed from the breast (on the pancreas meridian).

Although there are numerous problems relating

to the heart meridian, I believe the main cause is on the stomach and spleen/pancreas meridians – obvious in the problems with the menstrual cycle, cysts, bunions and appendectomy. The liver and gall bladder are also penetrated by the stomach meridian which could produce the symptoms of nausea and migraines. Note also that the kidneys are on the stomach meridian and the heart is on the kidney meridian. To care for a weak heart, do not overload the kidneys. This can be prevented by ensuring correct acid/alkaline balance in the stomach.

SMALL INTESTINE MERIDIAN

Female: Age – early 30s

Symptoms: Severe neck, back and shoulder problems – pinched sensation from shoulder down the arm – at one point lost all feeling in her arm; weak stomach – often experiences cramps after meals; weakness in throat; tennis elbow; at the age of six had a hernia in the groin; at age five suffered a severe ear infection which caused balance problems.

Problems along the small intestine meridian are obvious in these symptoms on the shoulder, neck/arm, elbow, ears and throat. Again, remember that meridians in the arms do not penetrate any major organs and one would have to look for the cause on one of the main meridians and the related organs. The weak stomach and cramps after meals indicate a stomach imbalance. The ch'i energy congestions are mainly located along the arm, shoulder, neck, ears and throat.

Male: Age – 30s

Symptoms: Extreme weakness and pain in his thigh muscles (quadriceps), causing the need for crutches. His GP had suggested hospitalization for traction, but he could not afford this treatment. He suffered mild but constant diarrhoea and a swollen stomach. The slightest movement caused palpitations. He lived on Coke and hamburgers.

This is a good example of a muscle imbalance. The quadriceps are related to the small intestine. As can be seen, he has a weak digestive system and very poor diet. The heart meridian is the partner, disease here manifesting as palpitations.

Colic

When a child is born, there are often complications during the birth process and the doctor may find it necessary to use forceps to guide the head through the birth canal. If you note where the small intestine meridian runs on the head, you will notice this is exactly where the forceps are usually placed. This exerts undue pressure on the head and therefore on this meridian, which can be the cause of colic in young babies. The twisting action which helps guide the baby through the birth canal can also twist the spine and result in a slight structural spinal defect.

To test whether the child has obstructions along the spine, hold the child upside down, with a firm grasp around both ankles. If there are no spinal defects, the child's back will be straight, with the arms out-stretched on either side. If the child hangs at a slight angle, this indicates a spinal defect which will require the attention of a good chiropractor. Once the spine is corrected, colic problems should diminish.

BLADDER MERIDIAN

Male: Age – 30s

Symptoms: This young runner suffered from extremely painful spurs on both heels. Other symptoms included a sore groin, lower back pain, spastic colon, headaches, and internal bleeding in the anal canal. He also felt gout symptoms in his feet after running.

Previous Operations: Appendectomy, tonsillectomy; operation on anal canal to stop bleeding.

The heel spurs were located on the lower back reflex, close to the bladder and rectum reflexes. The bladder meridian relates to headaches, lower back and rectum problems. The stomach meridian is evident in the operations and spastic colon. The excess uric acid evident in the post-run gout also indicates stomach imbalance.

Female: Age – late 40s

Symptoms: Sharp pains in both little toes; recent severe bladder infection for which she was prescribed antibiotics. Her eyes were weakening – she needed stronger glasses – and she suffered back problems. Ten years previously she had had a thrombosis in the back of the leg. She was constipated and often had stomach cramps. Rich foods made her nauseous. She had problems with menstrual cycle in her youth and went through troublesome menopause.

Previous Operations: Tonsillectomy, veins removed from left groin; adenoid operation.

The pains in the little toes indicated an imbalance in the bladder meridian. The bladder infections, weak eyes, back problems and thrombosis are further evidence of this congestion. Other meridians involved are the stomach and spleen/pancreas.

Female: Age – late 50s

Symptoms: Extremely swollen left leg particularly in the ankle area. Pain from the leg caused her to wake at night. She also suffered kidney and bladder problems – had difficulty passing water. She had kidney problems with each pregnancy. Angina was diagnosed by her GP.

Previous Operations: Ureter operations every two years until 1984; hysterectomy due to heavy periods; hernia; tonsillectomy; appendectomy; haemorrhoids; back operation in 1974 on third, fourth and fifth lumbar vertebrae.

The nerves radiating from the third, fourth and fifth lumbar vertebrae relate to the bladder, leg and ankle amongst other organs. Furthermore, the bladder meridian penetrates the same vertebrae. Obviously the cause of the kidney and bladder problems had never been solved, so these congestions now manifested in swollen legs. The heart is on the kidney meridian – relating to the angina diagnosis. The back pain and haemorrhoids are on the bladder meridian. Most operations occurred on the stomach and spleen/pancreas meridians.

KIDNEY MERIDIAN

Male: Age – mid 60s

Symptoms: General bad circulation, painful calves, tingling burning sensation in the feet. Has to get up every night to urinate.

Previous Operations: Three bypass operations; lumpectomy on the elbow.

Refer to the kidney meridian and note that the heart is situated on its pathway. The burning area on the feet was around the kidney reflexes. Furthermore, five plantar warts were situated on the heart reflex of his foot. The lump on the elbow was traced to the heart meridian. The calf muscles relate to the kidney's partner meridian, the bladder.

Female: Age – 37

Symptoms: Swollen ankles, oedema in the legs, spasms in the muscles around the hip bone when sitting incorrectly, lower back problems in thoracic vertebra number 11 (specified in an X-ray), genetic tendency to a weak heart condition, shortness of breath, pins and needles around the heart when there is an oxygen shortage.

The ankles, oedema and hip muscles are all examples of problems relating to the kidney meridian. The eleventh thoracic vertebra relates to the kidney. The heart is on the kidney meridian.

PERICARDIUM MERIDIAN

I have only seen symptoms along the pericardium meridian as part of larger case histories. Lesser symptoms such as eczema, psoriasis, pains in the armpits, carpal tunnel syndrome and arthritis in the middle finger have all been peripheral problems of imbalances along the stomach, spleen/pancreas or kidney meridians. Other symptoms indicative of an imbalance on this meridian are heart disease, disturbance in heart rhythm, mental disorders such as fear, nervousness and schizophrenia, car sickness and nausea.

TRIPLE BURNER MERIDIAN

Female: Age – early 30s

Symptoms: Severe eczema on both ring fingers – cannot wear rings. Prolapsed uterus – doctor recommended a hysterectomy after a difficult birth.

Previous Operations: Tonsillectomy; appendectomy; lumpectomy on breast around the nipple area.

All the symptoms and operations result from imbalances along the stomach and spleen/pancreas meridians. The effects of the imbalance had appeared as severe eczema on the ring fingers – the triple burner meridian.

Female: Age – early 40s

Symptoms: Pains around the ears – diagnosed by her GP as gout – had been so severe she was not able to wash or comb her hair or lie on her ear, particularly during menstruation or ovulation. She had menstrual cycle problems, sore breasts, and weakness in the throat.

This client drank red wine with her meals every evening which affected the triple burner meridian so severely that it resulted in gout. Menstrual cycle problems relate to the spleen/pancreas meridian, and the sore breast and weakness in the throat relate to its partner, the stomach meridian.

GALL BLADDER MERIDIAN

Female: Age – 30s

Symptoms: Migraine headaches behind the eyes and in the temples, coupled with nausea. Stiff shoulder joints and sensitive arm joints. Had a normal menstrual cycle but felt nauseous and bloated during menstruation. Suffers from sinus, post-nasal drip, eczema on hands, wrists and shins.

Migraine headaches and shoulder problems are on the gall bladder meridian. Nausea arises due to an imbalance in the liver/gall bladder. The sinus and post-nasal drip can be traced to the stomach meridian. Eczema on the shins relates to the pancreas meridian, and on the hands and wrist to the pericardium meridian.

Female: Age – 40s

Symptoms: Pains in the joints which had increased in severity over the years. Stomach easily upset, cannot eat rich foods, sensitive to wheat and dairy products. Palpitations. Still feels ovulation even though she has had a hysterectomy. Since a knee operation she has suffered inflammation in the hip, and both shoulders are very sensitive.

Previous Operations: Hysterectomy; operation on lateral side of the knee.

The knee operation cut right through the gall bladder meridian, and as the cause was not dealt with, the congestion 'moved' up to the hips and shoulders – both on the gall bladder meridian. Bile produced by the gall bladder helps digest fats, thus her aversion to rich foods also indicates gall bladder imbalance. Even though the most obvious problems are related to the gall bladder and its meridian, again the stomach meridian must be taken into account. The excess acidity in the body manifested as joint pains. The stomach meridian penetrates the gall bladder.

LIVER MERIDIAN

Female: Age – 8

Symptoms: She suffered severe candida problems (vaginal thrush) from the age of four. Doctors had prescribed creams and medication but nothing had helped. She had become introverted and developed social problems as a result of this affliction. Other symptoms included eczema on the inner thighs, chest weakness, nappy rash as a baby, numerous liver spots on the face and neck, and pain on the stomach meridian.

All these symptoms indicated unsolved problems with the stomach and its meridian. The stomach meridian runs through the liver, and the ch'i imbalance manifested on the liver meridian around the sexual region and the inner thigh area.

Female: Age – 50s

Symptoms: Low libido since hysterectomy two years previously, skin problems, weak bladder, eyes had weakened since a bladder repair operation.

The libido and hysterectomy are related to an imbalance on the liver meridian, but the hysterectomy could be related to the spleen/ pancreas. Notice the link between the eyes and the bladder.

Young Couple

This couple came into the clinic as they had an infertility problem. His symptoms were gout, low sperm count and jaundice a year earlier. Her symptoms were menstrual cycle problems and difficulty with ovulation. Most of her problems were along the stomach meridian and his along the liver meridian. Their daily intake of acidic foods was high, for example grains, meat, coffee, tea and soft drinks. Although they exhibited different symptoms, the main cause of their problems was stomach acidity.

Conclusion

In the past decade, reflexology has carved a respected niche for itself in the realm of holistic healing techniques. No longer is it a strange fringe practice ascribed to only by off-beat wierdos. People of all ages and from all walks of life have discovered the positive effects to be derived from foot therapy. The increasing demand for reflexology is proof of its burgeoning popularity and the pace at which reflexology has been, and is, expanding throughout the Western world is proof of its efficacy. The main objective of reflexology is to help people attain and maintain a better state of health and well-being. It does not promise to be a magic panacea for all ills, but there can no longer be any doubt that reflexology has an important role to play in the future of healthcare world-wide.

The remarkable results attained through reflexology stem from the amazing therapeutic potential present in the feet. Many reflexologists recommend stimulating hand reflexes as well as foot reflexes. Reflexes of body parts are mapped out on the hands in a fashion similar to those on the feet. Massaging the hands may elicit some positive effect, but nothing as powerful as the effect of foot massage. The reason for this, as has been explained in this book, is the fact that the six main meridians – those that actually penetrate major organs, the stomach, spleen/pancreas, liver, gall bladder, kidney and bladder meridians – all begin or end in the toes. The meridians represented in the hands – the heart, small intestine, circulation, triple burner, large intestine and lungs, although associated with specific organs (apart from the triple burner and circulation), do not actually penetrate any organs.

Hands, like feet, may be afflicted by deformities, but this is due largely to arthritic complaints. Often the same fingers on both hands will be afflicted – for example, the index fingers. All problems on the hands, like warts, eczema and nail problems, should be seen as an imbalance along a meridian. As the six main meridians do not penetrate any major organs – only sensory organs in the facial area – the imbalances which manifest on the hands should be seen as the result of congestions relating to the major organs and their meridians.

When the concept of the five elements is

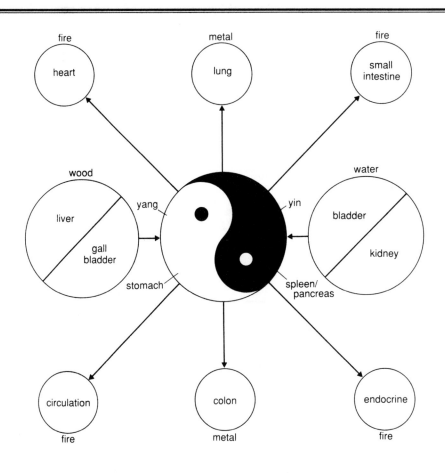

Fig. 99

introduced, the scenario becomes even more interesting. The six meridians in the hands are related to two elements – fire and metal. The fire element is represented in the heart meridian, small intestine meridian, circulation meridian and triple burner meridian; and the metal element in the large intestine and lung meridians. The six meridians in the feet represent the wood element in the liver and gall bladder meridians; the water element in the kidney and bladder meridians; and the earth element in the stomach and spleen/pancreas meridians.

When we correlate the elements with body functions and nutrition, the importance of correct nourishment becomes even more evident. The earth is central to our physical existence. We derive all physical nourishment from Mother Earth. Internally, the stomach and spleen/pancreas are the equivalent of the earth. To more fully understand this theory refer to the illustration in Figure 99. You will notice that I have placed the earth element in the centre to relate to the yin/yang symbol of perfect balance. The meridians related to the earth element are the stomach and spleen/pancreas. The stomach and its meridian control digestion, and the spleen and pancreas and their combined meridian control the distribution of ch'i energy released from food when it is digested. As has been mentioned in the section on meridians, if the stomach does not hold and digest food, the spleen cannot transform it and transport its essence. They are interdependent meridians, and work together more closely than any of the other meridians.

Earth is special among the elements, because she is the source of them, the centre from which they arise – as is the planet earth to our physical existence. Each of the elements is in constant relationship with the earth element, coming to life and dying within her realm. It has been written that the earth is both womb and tomb, the beginning and the end in the neverending cycle of life, death and rebirth.

Within earth we find water – the rivers, seas, springs; metal in the forms of minerals, gems and fuel (coal); and wood in the plant life. Relating this to meridians – the stomach meridian (earth) **penetrates the liver (wood), the kidneys (water)** and the lungs and large intestine (metal).

If you refer again to the illustration you will see the wood element on the left side of the earth, and water on the right side. To balance the earth element, we must have the correct nutrition from the plant kingdom – the wood element. Plants which have absorbed goodness from the earth and flourished in sunlight are imbued with vital ch'i energy, providing foods which are easy to digest and distribute. We must also have the correct quantity and quality of liquid – the water element – for the digestion and absorption of the food.

In the process of digesting food, some chemicals are released in the form of gases. This relates to the lungs – the metal element. Other ingredients will be transformed by the large intestine – again the metal element. In the illustration, the metal element is divided, one above and one below, as one metal element organ, the lungs, is concerned with deriving ch'i from air and gases; the other, the large intestine derives ch'i from food.

Energy is created by combustion, which releases pure ch'i from the impure. Here we find the correlation with the fire element of the small intestine. Ch'i is further transported via the circulation, assisted by the heart and the endocrine system – these three meridians also belong to the fire element. In the illustration, the fire element has been divided into four to represent the related meridians.

This description of the five elements has been included to provide some food for thought and to further elucidate the theories contained in this book. It emphasizes the relevance of the theory that the potent positive effects derived from reflexology are linked to the presence of meridians in the feet – meridians that relate to the three central elements of earth, wood and water, and which all penetrate the major body organs, whose functions are specifically associated with nutrition, digestion and distribution. Applying therapeutic pressure to the feet stimulates not only the reflexes and related body parts, but also the six main meridians, thereby helping to clear congestions along the meridians and activate the circulation of vital ch'i energy, which revitalizes the whole body.

Reflexology is an extremely effective holistic therapy, the positive effects of which can only be enhanced by any other holistic therapy, attitude and activity. Many different factors influence each individual, and therefore affect his ability to assimilate and respond to the healing process. Numerous conditions have an effect on our being – some within our control, some beyond our control. In order to help offset the negative effects of conditions we cannot control, such as the earth's gravity, the movement of the sun, moon and stars, global and social pressures, and climate, we should make more effort to alter those conditions we are able to change in order to improve our quality of life. The things we can do for ourselves may require some discipline and effort, but they will make an enduring and worthwhile contribution towards attaining perfect health.

One factor within our control which has a

profound effect on health is diet. Referring to the theory examined in this chapter, the earth element (relating to the stomach and spleen/pancreas) is central to health. Adopting a healthy diet can work wonders in helping to eliminate disease, as the root cause of numerous diseases can be linked to incorrect nutrition. Many conditions cannot be treated 100 per cent effectively unless modifications are made to the diet. A good practitioner will usually enquire about diet and encourage necessary modifications.

Relaxation techniques are also beneficial as an adjunct to reflexology. Stress is another major cause of disease, so anything which helps alleviate stress is worth pursuing. Possible options are T'ai Chi Chu'an, yoga and meditation as well as breathing and visualization techniques. Some form of more vigorous exercise such as aerobics, swimming, jogging or gym is also recommended, to offset the negative effects of sedentary living common in the modern world. Physical exercise activates the circulation which in turn encourages the body to function more efficiently.

As reflexology is a holistic therapy, it can be effectively and successfully combined with other holistic therapies. These include Bach Flower Remedies, herbal treatment, naturopathy, Ayurvedic medicine, homoeopathy, hydrotherapy and acupuncture, as well as any form of massage such as shiatsu and aromatherapy. However, moderation is the key. Adopting too many therapies is not recommended, Whatever the choice, the goal of all holistic therapies is the same – to stimulate the body's own inherent healing potential in a natural and safe way, in order to assist in alleviating the suffering of those afflicted by disease.

Reflexology helps us to attune to our bodies and to understand ourselves as part of a greater whole . . . to tune in to the natural laws of the cosmos and work towards a more holistic approach to life – an approach that results in a balanced and fulfilled existence. Perfect health requires discipline and energy, but the effort pays good dividends. A productive, healthy and fulfilled existence *is* within reach. It is not necessary to suffer through life, riddled with pain and disease. And we need look no further than to our feet for relief. If we take care of our feet, they will take care of us and the rewards can be remarkable. We can then say to our feet, with genuine gratitude; 'Thanks for the support!'

APPENDIX

The VacuFlex Reflexology System

The VacuFlex Reflexology System evolved from an idea I first came upon in Denmark. Over a period of twelve years, I have developed and systemized this approach to reflexology in order to modernize the practice.

The full VacuFlex treatment is a two-phase treatment which combines the stimulation of the foot reflexes with rebalancing of the meridians. This system is often referred to as the 'boot' system due to the large spacesuit-like felt boots used on the feet. The VacuFlex system combines three alternative therapies – reflexology, acupressure and cupping. This combination has proved to be very effective in relieving problems otherwise difficult to combat, such as back problems, strokes, circulation problems and arthritis.

Vacuum therapy is acknowledged as an ancient treatment, having been practised since primitive times when animal horns were used as cups. Cups made from burnt clay were discovered in ancient Mesopotamia. In Greece these cups were made of bronze, while other examples have been found constructed of brass, porcelain and glass. The VacuFlex cups, referred to as 'pads', are made of silicone.

Needles, lasers, finger pressure or suction pads placed on specific meridian points stimulate related nerves which transmit electrical impulses to the spinal cord and brain. The suction pressure increases the flow of blood and oxygen to congested areas, causing toxic stagnation to disperse. The pressure also encourages tissue and muscle regeneration by stimulating blood supply and nutrients to the affected areas.

The VacuFlex boots come in two sizes, adults and children. These plastic covered boots, which are connected to a vacuum pump, are placed on the feet. Air is suctioned from the boot to create a uniform pressure over the entire foot, which stimulates all the reflexes. This provides a full reflexology treatment in just five minutes. The pressure can be controlled, and a reading is possible on the pressure gauge.

The pressure from the boots leaves a map of colours on the feet for approximately 15 seconds. These colours relate to the reflexes that would have been sore or sensitive during a manual massage. The colours are blue, red, yellow and white, depending on the severity of the problem. These colours change from treatment to treatment in accordance with the healing process.

The solar plexus, known as the abdominal brain because it contains so many nerves and nerve networks, is also stimulated by the boots during the first stage of treatment with the result that spasms and cramps cannot occur. It is for this reason that the system was found to be particularly beneficial in its original development to help a spastic epileptic child who had suffered cramps and spasms with conventional reflexology.

It is often assumed that the pressure exerted by the boots is stronger than the thumb pressure techniques. This is not so. A test conducted by an engineer proved that the pressure applied using the central portion of the tip of the thumb exerts 5.29 times more pressure than the lowest scale of the VacuFlex System, which ranges from 40 to 80 kilopascals. The difference is that the boots apply uniform, constant and continuous pressure for a period of five minutes, while the thumb pressure is not uniform or constant.

The second stage of the treatment involves stimulating some of the strategic acupuncture points along the meridians and the arms and legs. This is applied with the suction pads operated by the same vacuum system as the boots.

Some people feel the use of mechanical equipment diminishes the interaction between client and practitioner. This is not necessarily so. The vital energy exchange is still apparent as the movement of the pads is very physical. Also, the treatment should always be completed with hand-executed relaxation techniques described earlier in the book. People generally find the boot less painful than hand massage, and children can be treated comfortably with this system. The thoroughness of the VacuFlex system ensures that the client always receives a complete and effective treatment irrespective of the practitioner's accuracy.

This system has proved successful in alleviating a wide range of disorders. To verify the accuracy of this treatment, a research study was conducted in Britain by Carol Bosiger, a member of the South African Reflexology Society and founder of the Association of VacuFlex Reflexologists in Britain. It was published in the *Journal of Alternative and Complementary Medicine*, August 1989. Back pain was chosen for this study because it is a common problem, often with no apparent cause or remedy, for which VacuFlex has been found to be particularly effective.

The subjects were eleven patients from four practitioners in Britain. The patients were aged 31–56 and presented predominantly with back pain during the twelve months ending October 1988. The aim of the study was to determine the degree of success achieved by VacuFlex in removing their symptoms after one to ten treatments. In each case the treatment involved weekly sessions lasting 30 minutes.

CASE HISTORIES

Miss C from Isle of Sheppey, aged 46.
Severe lower back pain for nearly ten months which was not due to any injury. GP told her that she would have to live with the pain. Physiotherapy did not help. After two treatments pain totally ceased. She has had no recurrence since.

Mr T from Isle of Sheppey, aged 50.
Diagnosed by his GP as having a whiplash injury. One treatment gave total relief.

Mrs MC from Isle of Sheppey, aged 52.
Severe sciatica for two years. Shoulder and hip pain which had been diagnosed as arthritis. She took painkillers regularly and had to roll out of bed. After the first treatment the pain had lessened. After the third treatment the pain had gone and she was able to get out of bed normally.

Mrs C from Isle of Sheppey, aged 50.
Had to rely on painkillers for constant lower back pain which had been present for eight years. She also suffered shoulder and knee pains and very heavy periods. The first treatment resulted in immediate relief from back pain and the patient was able to bend down to replace her stockings.

At the second treatment she reported the shoulder pain had cleared but there was pain in her right knee. For the first time in her life she had a painless period. Colon and bladder were more active. By the tenth treatment had a feeling of 'great well-being' and was pain-free.

Mrs D from London, aged 52.

Constant back pain and hardly able to move after gardening. Pain worse on wakening. Irritable bowel for three years. Hiatus hernia with heartburn and acidity. Neck and shoulders very stiff. Worn glasses for forty years. Occasional headaches. After the first treatment the back was improved and diarrhoea ceased. Feeling tired. During the following three treatments the back pain became worse and then more localized. At the tenth treatment, the back pain had gone as had all digestive problems. Energy was very high, and she was sleeping better than for several years.

Mr S from London, aged 31.

Pain in lower back so bad he could hardly stand at times. Left knee, which had been broken three years previously, was very painful. Receiving medication for acidic stomach. Extremely sensitive feet, tickle in throat, extremely cold, very tired. All improved each week of treatment. By fourth treatment was training without strapping injured knee. At sixth and final treatment great energy and no pains or problems.

Mr T from London, aged 56.

Pain in lower back for ten years, unable to straighten after sitting. Tried numerous therapies without finding relief. Fibrositis in left shoulder twenty years ago not causing current problem. Two pulmonary embolisms twenty and ten years ago. Sleeping badly. At the end of first treatment considerable relief of back pain. At second treatment reported back pain nearly gone, twinges in left shoulder, sleeping greatly improved. At sixth treatment reported all pain gone and sleeping well. Great energy.

Mrs R from London, aged 42.

Neck spasms and stiffness, tense shoulders, lower back pain with associated leg and knee pain. Extreme tiredness, sensitive eyes, tinnitus in left ear, sore throat, easily out of breath, stiff arms, cramps in legs and toes, coughing up foul phlegm, heartburn, wind, acidity, migraine, severe PMT with bloating, painful breasts, exhaustion and depression, heavy painful periods, overweight. Terrible pains in solar plexus area. Underwent hospital tests which revealed nothing.

At second treatment solar plexus tender, ears clearer, felt lighter, jaw firmer, more relaxed and neck easier. At third treatment no headaches, calm, slight sore throat, neck fine, skin softer, ankles swollen, arms more relaxed and back improved. At fourth treatment knees and legs sore, breasts down one cup-size, glands sore and throat rough, swollen ankles improved, lost 7lb. At next treatment had experienced pain – and clot-free period with no PMT, totally pain-free breasts, throat still rough, neck, legs and ankles fine. At eighth treatment had totally unnoticeable period, very supple, no phlegm, lovely skin, energy great, all aches and pains gone.

Mrs P from Essex, aged 53.

Extreme pains in lower back, especially at night which prevented sleep. Pain started in lumbar region, spread up spine to shoulders, unable to turn over in bed. Stiff neck and shoulders, arthritis in knees, heavy painful legs, swollen ankles and feet, stiff hands and fingers. Water retention and overweight since childhood, tension headaches, eyes sensitive to light and sore, constipation and weak bladder. Very tired. At second treatment reported loss of 1lb, one bad headache, neck and shoulders painful on left side, slept better but back still painful during day, knees improved to point where kneeling possible, hands and fingers stiff, more energy. At third treatment lost further 2lb, more energy, yellow vaginal discharge, no headaches, eyes less red, neck and shoulders improved, lower back improved and sleep much improved. Hands and fingers same. General improvements but roving aches and pains until ninth treatment when eyes were clear, no discomfort or redness, legs and feet comfortable with no swelling, further 8lb weight loss, shoulders and neck easier. For first time in years sleeping all night, far more supple, more energy.

Miss K from London, aged 39.

Lower back pain, stiff neck and shoulders, weak right ankle, knees crack, stomach pains since teens, bloating and acidity. Very hyped-up, bouts of anxiety, eyes very itchy for two years, with skin around eyes sore, dry and cracked, eyes puffy in mornings and weepy. Ears itchy and weepy, and 'pop' often. Itchy red patches on cheeks and forehead. Weak bladder, up several times at night, cramps in legs, bad PMT getting worse.

At second treatment reported eyes very sore and itchy, very tired and depressed, stomach improved. At third treatment eyes still sore, not tired or depressed, stomach pain gone, back, neck and shoulders no pain. Bad taste in mouth, feeling like a 'different person'. At fourth treatment PMT bad, eyes itchy but skin much improved, no patches, no itching. At fifth treatment heavier, longer period, eyes improved, skin very good, feeling of energy.

Patient then had four-week break. At next treatment reported light problem-free period with no PMT. Eyes still improving and more relaxed. After two more treatments all problems gone, eyes sparkling, skin clear, no aches or pains, great energy.

Mr T from London, aged 32.

Stiff neck with headaches starting in neck, lower back pain when lifting. Gallstones diagnosed two years earlier, eyes tired, eyeballs twitched spasmodically, dermatitis, tinnitus in left ear, heartburn, loose stools, stomach pains. Sore red patches on cheeks and forehead, very tired especially after last six months.

At second treatment reported headaches, feeling tired, very shaky, eyes very sore and tired. Flashing lights improved, neck sore. No heartburn, stomach improved. Skin worse, lower back improved, sleeping more deeply. At third treatment no headaches, not as tired, no shaking, eyes fine, neck fine, bowels improved, skin great deal better, lower back improved. By fifth treatment able to start running again, very calm, energy good, aches and pains gone, concentration improved.

Conclusion

The study showed that all types of back pain responded quickly to VacuFlex with total relief in all eleven cases after one to ten treatments. The treatment also successfully alleviated a wide range of additional related and non-related complaints experienced by the patient (which is a normal response to reflexology generally). It is a pleasant and gentle therapy which is suitable for most sensitive patients.

For further information contact:
Inge Dougans
PO Box 68283
Bryanston
Johannesburg 2021
South Africa

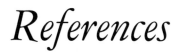

References

INTRODUCTION

1 Robert Becker MD and Gary Seldon. *The Body Electric*. p19.
2 Patrick Holford. 'Pollution Protection': *Here's Health* magazine, August 1989, p14.
3 *ibid*, p15.
4 Andrew Stanway MB, MRCP. *Alternative Medicine*. p36.
5 Geoff Pike. *The Power of Ch'i*. p9.
6 D. & J. Lawson-Wood. *Five Elements of Acupuncture & Chinese Massage*. pp70 & 20.
7 Philippa Mckinley. 'Secrets of the Life Force'. *Here's Health* magazine, January 1991, p11, 12.
8 Ted J. Kaptchuk OMD. *The Web That Has No Weaver*. p8.
9 Robert Becker, pp79–80.
10 Lyall Watson. *Beyond Supernature*. pp92–7.
11 *ibid*
12 *ibid*
13 John Davidson. *Subtle Energy*. p19.
14 *ibid*, pp122–3.
15 Lyall Watson. *Supernature 11*. p105.
16 Lyall Watson. *Beyond Supernature*. p102.

SECTION 1: CHAPTER 1 HISTORY

1 Michelle Arnot. *Foot Notes*. pp8–9.
2 *ibid*, p26.
3 *ibid*, p21.
4 *ibid*, pxx.
5 *ibid*, p28.
6 *ibid*, p30.
7 Christine Issel. *Reflexology: Art, Science and History*. pp8–9.
8 *ibid*, pp 38–39.
9 Harry Bond Bressler. *Zone Therapy*. p29.
10 Issel, pp30–31.
11 *ibid*, p35.
12 *ibid*, pp24–5.
13 Ann Gillanders. *Reflexology – The Ancient Answer to Modern Ailments*. p35.
14 William H. Fitzgerald and Edwin F. Bowers. *Zone Therapy*. p9.
15 Issel, p52.
16 Dwight C. Byers. *Better Health with Foot Reflexology*. p3.
17 Issel, pp54–5.
18 Byers, p5.
19 Issel, p63.
20 Issel, p120–21.
21 Gillanders, p13.

SECTION 1: CHAPTER 2 WHAT IS REFLEXOLOGY AND HOW DOES IT WORK?

1 Issel, p122.
2 Kevin and Barbara Kunz. *The Complete Guide to Foot Reflexology*. p2.
3 Gillanders, p25.
4 Doreen Bayley. *Reflexology Today*. p13.
5 Eunice D. Ingham. *Stories The Feet Have Told Thru Reflexology*. p10.
6 Kunz, p16.
7 Issel, p114.
8 Issel, p75.
9 Kunz, p17.
10 Issel, p119.
11 *ibid*, pp117–18.
12 *ibid*, p77.
13 Omraam Mikhaël Aïvanhov. *the zodiac, key to man and to the universe*. pp79–80.
14 *ibid*, pp83–9.
15 *ibid*, pp92–6.

SECTION 2 THE HOLISTIC APPROACH

1 Dr E. Cheraskin and Dr W. M. Ringsdorf Jr with Arline Brecher. *Psychodietetics*. p15.
2 Franklyn Sills. *The Polarity Process*. p87.
3 Davidson, p126.
4 Cheraskin, p17.
5 Lyall Watson. *Beyond Supernature*. p117.
6 Harold Saxton Burr. *Blueprint for Immortality*. p12.
7 Deepak Chopra MD *Perfect Health*. p12.
8 Burr, p13.
9 Sills, p91.

SECTION 2: CHAPTER 1 ENERGIES

1 Becker, p247.
2 Lyall Watson. *Gifts of Unknown Things*. p105.
3 Becker, p249.
4 *ibid*, p255.
5 Burr, p14.
6 Lyall Watson. *Supernature*. p52.
7 Becker, p244–5.
8 Lyall Watson. *Supernature*. p47.
9 Juliet Brooke Ballard. *The Hidden Laws of the Earth*. p100.
10 Lyall Watson. *Supernature*. p50.
11 Becker, p275.
12 *ibid*, p272.
13 *ibid*, p278.
14 *ibid*, p285.

15 *ibid*, pp302–3.
16 Davidson, pp119–20.
17 *ibid*, p117–18.
18 Becker, p291.
19 *ibid*, p277.
20 *ibid*, p313.
21 *ibid*, p327.
22 *ibid*, p327.

SECTION 2: CHAPTER 2 STRESS

1 Laura Norman with Thomas Cowan. *Feet First*. p130.
2 Becker, p292.
3 Cheraskin p.17
4 Alvin Toffler. *Future Shock*.

SECTION 2: CHAPTER 3 DIET

1 Ballard, pp82–3.
2 Cheraskin, p28.
3 Holford, p13.
4 Dr George Lewith & Dr Julian Kenyon. *Clinical Ecology*. p63.
5 Holford, p13.

SECTION 3: CHAPTER 6 FOOT CARE

1 Arnot, p3.
2 *ibid*, p166–77.

SECTION 4 THE PRINCIPLES OF CHINESE MEDICINE

1 Kaptchuk, p51.
2 Ilza Veith. *The Yellow Emperor's Classic of Internal Medicine*. p105.
3 *ibid*, p220.
4 John Blofeld. *Taoism* . p3.
5 *ibid*, pp2–3.
6 Veith, pp115–23.
7 Chee Soo. *The Taoist Ways of Healing*. p23.
8 Veith, p17.
9 Chee Soo, p24.
10 Veith, p19.
11 Chee Soo, p93.
12 Stephen T. Chang. *The Complete System of Chinese Self-Healing*. p32.
13 McKinley, *Here's Health* magazine. p11.
14 Chee Soo, pp26–7.
15 Veith, pp152–3.
16 Veith, pp104–5.

SECTION 4: CHAPTER 1 THE FIVE ELEMENTS

1 Lawson-Wood, p40.
2 Yoshio Manaka MD and Ian A. Urquhart PhD. *The Layman's Guide to Acupuncture*. pp39–40.

3 Gillanders, p12.
4 Lawson-Wood, p40.
5 Dianne M. Connelly PhD, Mac. *Traditional Acupuncture: The Law of the Five Elements*. p27.
6 *ibid*, p26.
7 *ibid*, p25.
8 Veith, p109.
9 Connelly, p22.
10 *ibid*, p23.
11 Mark Seem PhD with Joan Kaplan *Bodymind Energetics*. pp 93–4.
12 *ibid*,. pp93–4.
13 Connelly, p21.
14 Seem, p85.
15 Connelly, p53.
16 Seem, p87.
17 Connelly, pp51–2.
18 *ibid*, pp63–5.
19 *ibid*, pp63–4.
20 *ibid*, p63.
21 Seem, p90.
22 Connelly, p75.
23 Seem, p92.
24 Connelly, p80.

SECTION 4: CHAPTER 2
MERIDIANS

1 Bruce Copen PhD, DLitt. *The Magic of the Aura*. pp29–30.
2 John F. Thie. *Touch for Health*. p17.
3 Chee Soo, p94.
4 Dr Michael Nightingale. *Acupuncture*. pp51–2.
5 Veith, p30.
6 *ibid*, pp25–8.
7 Kaptchuk, p53.
8 *ibid*, p43.
9 Veith, pp30–34.
10 *ibid*, p28.
11 Kaptchuk, p53.
12 Veith, p133.
13 Thie, pp18–19.
14 Nightingale, p61.
15 *ibid*, pp73–4.
16 Kaptchuk, p78.
17 Janet Riddle, *Anatomy and Physiology Applied to Nursing*. p.51.

18 Veith, p133.
19 *ibid*, p139.
20 Iona Marsaa-Teegurden. *Handbook of Acupressure II*. p10.
21 Katpchuk, p56.
22 *ibid*, pp56–7.
23 Thie, p96.
24 *ibid*, p98.
25 *ibid*, p100.
26 *ibid*, p102.
27 Veith, p133.
28 Marsaa-Teegurden, p10.
29 Thie, p104.
30 *ibid*, p106.
31 *ibid*, p108.
32 Veith, p133.
33 *ibid*, p139.
34 Connelly, p54.
35 Kaptchuk, pp57–68.
36 Connelly, p54.
37 Thie, p36.
38 *ibid*, p38.
39 *ibid*, p40.
40 *ibid*, p42.
41 Veith, p133.
42 Marsaa-Teegurden, and Kaptchuk, p58.
43 Kaptchuk, pp58–9.
44 Thie, p44.
45 *ibid*, p46.
46 *ibid*, p48.
47 *ibid*, p50.
48 Veith, p133.
49 *ibid*, p139.
50 Marsaa-Teegurden, p12.
51 Kaptchuk, p54, and Marsaa-Teegurden, p16.
52 Kaptchuk, p54.
53 Thie, p52.
54 Veith, p133.
55 Marsaa-Teegurden p12.
56 Connelly, p37.
57 Thie, p54.
58 *ibid*, p56.
59 Veith, p133.
60 Marsaa-Teegurden, p20, and Kaptchuk, p68, and Connelly p78.
61 Thie, p58.
62 *ibid*, p60.

63 *ibid*, p62.
64 Veith, p133.
65 *ibid*, p139.
66 Kaptchuk, pp62–3.
67 Connelly, p77.
68 Marsaa-Teegurden, p22.
69 Thie, p64.
70 *ibid*, p66.
71 *ibid*, p68.
72 Marsaa-Teegurden, p25.
73 Thie, p70.
74 *ibid*, p72.
75 *ibid*, p74.
76 *ibid*, p76.
77 Veith, p133.
78 Marsaa-Teegurden, p26.
79 *ibid*, p26.
80 Thie, p78.
81 *ibid*, p80.
82 *ibid*, p82.
83 *ibid*, p84.
84 *ibid*, p86.
85 Veith, p133.
86 Marsaa-Teegurden, p28.
87 *ibid*, p28.
88 Kaptchuk, p66-7.
89 Thie, p88.
90 *ibid*, p90.
91 Veith, p133.
92 *ibid*, p139.
93 Kaptchuk, pp59–60.
94 Marsaa-Teegurden, p30.
95 Kaptchuk, p60, and Marsaa-Teegurden, p30.
96 Thie, p92.
97 *ibid*, p94.
98 Kaptchuk, p78.
99 Manaka p73.
100 Seem, p33.
101 Chinese Traditional Medical College p51, and Kaptchuk, p104.
102 Jorgen Frydenlund. *Meridianlaren* forlaget Alterna.
103 Thie, p34.
104 Seem, p33.
105 Chinese Traditional Medical College, p55, and Kaptchuk, p107.
106 Thie, p32.

Bibliography

Aïvanhov, Omraam Mikhaël. *the zodiac, key to man and to the universe*. Editions Prosveta, Fréjus, France, 1986.

Arnot, Michelle. *Foot Notes*. Sphere Books Ltd, 1982.

Ballard, Juliet Brooke *The Hidden Laws of the Earth*. A.R.E. Press, Virginia Beach, Virginia, 1986.

Bayley, Doreen. *Reflexology Today*. Thorsons, New York, 1986.

Becker, Robert, MD, and Seldon, Gary. *The Body Electric*. Quill, William Morrow, NewYork, 1985.

Blofeld, John. *Taoism – The Quest For Immortality*. Unwin Paperbacks, London, 1979.

Bressler, Harry Bond. *Zone Therapy*. Health Research, Mokelumne Hill, CA, 1971.

Burr, Harold Saxton. *Blueprint for Immortality*. The C. W. Daniel Company Limited, Saffron Walden, 1972.

Byers, Dwight C. *Better Health with Foot Reflexology*. Ingham Publishing, St Petersburg, Florida, 1986.

Cheraskin, E. and Ringsdorf Jr, W. M. with Brecher, Arline. *Psychodietetics*. Bantam Books, New York, 1985.

Chinese Traditional Medical College of Shanghai and Chinese Traditional Research Institute of Shanghai. *Anatomical Charts of the Acupuncture Points and 14 Meridians*. Shanghai People's Publishing House, 1976.

Chopra, Deepak, MD. *Perfect Health*. BantamBooks, Transworld Publishers, London, 1990.

Connelly, Dianne M. PhD, MAC *Traditional Acupuncture: The Law of the Five Elements*. The Centre for Traditional Acupuncture Inc., Columbia, Maryland, 1989.

Copen, Bruce, PhD, DLitt. *Magic of the Aura*. Academic Publications, Haywards Heath, 1976.

Davidson, John. *Subtle Energy*. The C. W. Daniel Company Limited, Saffron Walden, 1987.

Fast, Julius. *You and Your Feet*. Pelham Books, London, 1971.

Fitzgerald, William H., and Bowers, Edwin F *Zone Therapy*. Health Research, Mokelumne Hill, CA, 1917.

Frydenlund, Jorgen. *Meridianlaren* forlaget Alterna.

Gillanders, Ann. *Reflexology – The Ancient Answer to Modern Ailments*. Gillanders, 1987.

Goosman-Legger, Astrid. *Zone Therapy Using Foot Massage*. The C. W. Daniel Company Limited, Saffron Walden, 1983.

Gore, Anya. *Reflexology*. Optima, London, 1990.

Grinberg, Avi. *Holistic Reflexology*. Thorsons, Wellingborough, 1989.

Hall, Nicola M. *Reflexology – A Patient's Guide*. Thorsons, Wellingborough, 1986.

Hall, Nicola M. *Reflexology – A Way To Better Health*. Pan Books, London, 1988.

Holford, Patrick. 'Population Protection'. *Here's Health* magazine, August 1989.

Ingham, Eunice D. *Stories The Feet Can Tell Thru Reflexology*. Ingham Publishing, St. Petersburg, Florida, 1938.

Ingham, Eunice D. *Stories The Feet Have Told Thru Reflexology*. Ingham Publishing, St. Petersburg, Florida, 1951.

Issel, Christine. *Reflexology: Art, Science and History*. New Frontier Publishing, Sacramento, 1990.

Kaptchuk, Ted J., OMD. *The Web That Has No Weaver*. Congden & Weed, New York, 1983.

Kunz, Kevin and Barbara. *The Complete Guide to Foot Reflexology*. Thorsons, Wellingborough, 1982.

Lawson-Wood, D. & J. *The Five Elements of Acupuncture & Chinese Massage*. Health Science Press, Devon, 1985.

Lewith, George (M.D.) and Kenyon, Julian (M.D.). *Clinical Ecology*. Thorsons, Wellingborough, 1985.

Maarsa-Teegurden, Iona. *Handbook of Acupressure II*, Ginseng du Foundation, 1981.

MacDonald, Alexander. *Acupuncture – From Ancient Art to Modern Medicine* Unwin, London, 1982.

Majhisttagenmalm. *Zonterapi og Urtemeduim*. Komma Helse.

Manaka, Yoshio, MD, and Urquhart, Ian A., PhD.

A Layman's Guide to Acupuncture. Weatherhill, New York, 1972.

Mann, Felix. *Acupuncture*. Pan Books, London,1971.

Marquardt, Hanne. *Reflex Zone Therapy of the Feet*. Thorsons, Wellingborough, 1983.

McKinley, Philippa 'Secrets of the Life Force.' *Here's Health* magazine, January 1991.

Nightingale, Michael. *Acupuncture*. Optima, London, 1987.

Norman, Laura. *Feet First*. Simon & Schuster Inc., New York, 1988.

Pike, Geoff. *The Power of Ch'i*. Bay Books, Sydney, 1980.

Riddle, Janet. *Anatomy & Physiology Applied to Nursing*. Churchill Livingstone, Edinburgh, 1985.

Russel, Lewis, and Hardy, Bob. *Healthy Feet*. Optima, London, 1988.

Seem, Mark, PhD, with Kaplan, Joan. *Bodymind Energetics*. Thorsons, Wellingborough, 1987.

Sills, Franklyn. *The Polarity Process*. Element Books, Shaftesbury, 1989.

Soo, Chee. *The Taoist Ways of Healing*. Aquarian Press, Wellingborough, 1986.

Stanway, Dr Andrew. *Alternative Medicine – A Guide to Natural Therapies*. Penguin Books, Harmondsworth, 1982.

Thie, John F. *Touch For Health*. T. H. Enterprises, Pasadena, California, 1973.

Toffler, Alvin. *Future Shock*. The Bodley Head, London, 1975.

Veith, Ilza. *The Yellow Emperor's Classic of Internal Medicine*. University of California Press, 1972.

Wagner, Franz PhD. *Reflex Zone Massage*. Thorsons, Wellingborough, 1987.

Watson, Lyall. *Supernature*. Coronet Books, London, 1974.

Watson, Lyall. *Supernature II*. Sceptre, London, 1987.

Watson, Lyall. *Beyond Supernature*. Hodder & Stoughton, London, 1986.

Watson, Lyall. *The Romeo Error*. Anchor Press/ Doubleday, New York, 1974.

Watson Lyall. *Gifts of Unknown Things*. Sceptre, London, 1987.

Index